Preventing **Cancer** in a Toxic World

Your Health Press

Preventing **Cancer** in a Toxic World

Avoiding Risk, Reducing Risk and Optimizing Health

M. Sara Rosenthal, Ph.D.

Preventing Cancer in a Toxic World
Your Health Press
copyright© M. Sara Rosenthal and Your Health Press, 2012.

Important Notice:
The purpose of this book is to educate. It is sold with the understanding that the author and publisher shall have neither liability nor responsibility for any injury caused or alleged to be caused directly or indirectly by the information contained in this book. While every effort has been made to ensure its accuracy, the book's contents should not be construed as medical advice. Each person's health needs are unique. To obtain recommendations appropriate to your particular situation, please consult a qualified health care provider.

All trademarked products appear herein minus the registered trademark symbol.

Design of print and digital editions: Anita Janik-Jones
Cover photo: istockphoto.com
Interior images: morguefile.com

ISBN: 978-0-9859724-5-5

In memory of Megan Stendebach
October 21, 1961 – March 18, 2008

"What are the odds of one person getting struck by lightning three times?"
—Megan Stendebach, 2007

Megan was a friend I knew too briefly, diagnosed with thyroid cancer in
1997, breast cancer in 2006, and gastrointestinal cancer in 2008.

TABLE OF CONTENTS

ACKNOWLEDGMENTS

I wish to thank my colleagues at the University of Toronto Center for Health Promotion, who formed the Cancer Prevention Interest Group. Individuals who served as content experts for portions of this book include: Ellen J. Hahn, DNS, RN professor, University of Kentucky College of Nursing, Tobacco Policy Research Program director, Kentucky Center for Smoke-free Policy (reviewer for chapter 2); Heather Pierce, Ph.D., CGC, former director, Genetic Counseling Program, University of Kentucky (reviewer for genetics section of chapter 7); and Hollie Swanson, Ph.D., associate professor, Department of Molecular and Biomedical Pharmacology, University of Kentucky (reviewer for chapters 9 and 10).

I am grateful to Ellen Tulchinsky, the medical librarian who served as research assistant

PRIMARY PREVENTION IS "CANCER CONTRACEPTION"

Today, cancer is "controlled" through early detection, treatment, rehabilitation, and palliative care (which means symptom relief rather than curative treatment). These are not great ways to ultimately deal with the problem of cancer. What we really need to focus on "stopping cancer before it starts" (a term used in the world of primary prevention of cancer) or even, as one oncologist puts it: "cancer contraception." The term *primary prevention* refers to preventing a disease at its origins. There is a world of difference between the terms *prevention* and *detection*. There is also a vast difference between primary prevention and secondary prevention. When the medical community discusses cancer prevention, it usually means cancer detection through screening or other diagnostic tests, or by self-exam; meanwhile, prescribing drugs to prevent a certain cancer is a form of secondary prevention.

Primary prevention means changing the behavior that causes the disease or eliminating the carcinogen responsible for the disease. For example, if smoking is responsible for most lung cancers, not smoking can stop most lung cancer cases before they start. Lung cancer afflicting nonsmokers, however, is on the rise and certainly is linked to environmental tobacco smoke, although other carcinogens are also involved. Stopping secondhand, or environmental, tobacco smoke must be done through policy changes that you can participate in, but cannot completely control, other than avoiding smoke-filled areas, when possible. Certain occupations create exposures that you may not be able to avoid without changing occupations or dramatically changing the industries. Choices in foods, food preparation methods, personal household products, and toiletries may also affect exposures to certain chemicals and carcinogens.

Not all cancers are on the rise, however. We are beginning to see a reduction in the incidence and mortality of a few major cancers, including lung cancer in men, and stomach and colorectal cancer in both sexes. No one knows why we're seeing a decline in stomach cancer. (Over fifty years ago, stomach cancer was the most worrisome cancer in the world, and it has now fallen to eleventh place in North America for both sexes combined, due in large part to a decline in the consumption of preserved or pickled foods.) The decline in lung cancer in men is attributed to the more aggressive anti-smoking campaigns and the decline in colon cancer in both sexes is attributed to better education about fiber and high-fiber diets.

Because so many cancers are linked to a poor diet and sedentary living, by focusing on primary prevention programs aimed at stopping cancer before it starts, we can also help reduce the incidence of a number of the killer chronic diseases, such as heart disease or type 2 diabetes. By looking at environmental toxins, we may also be able to reduce the incidence of more mysterious environmental diseases, such as chronic fatigue syndrome (CFS) or multiple chemical sensitivity (MCS).

In order to prevent future cancers, we have to look at its natural history. Many cancers (including breast and stomach cancer) are influenced by events in childhood as well as later in life. Strategies we adopt today may take twenty to forty years to deliver a clear return or benefit. This is one of the reasons why it's been so difficult to convince governments to spend money on primary prevention programs, and why the bulk of research is going into secondary prevention, such as treatment or the identification of cancer genes. But that doesn't mean that delaying these initiatives makes sense; it means that the sooner we act, the sooner we can see the rewards.

The information in this book is not about conspiracy theories or unsupported facts. It is based on a careful review of the global and interdisciplinary cancer literature, representing a consensus of viewpoints. *In a nutshell, this book is based on what scientists can agree on.* The consensus of cancer researchers is that there is an alarming array of environmental causes of cancer that range from lifestyle and dietary factors within our control to environmental pollutants and carcinogens in our workplaces and beyond (much of which is beyond our immediate control), as well as genetic mutations—many of which may be turned on by various environmental triggers and personal behaviors. Also included in this book are recommendations and suggestions made in collaboration with experts in cancer prevention and toxicology.

The information contained in this book is supported by accepted scientific evidence and studies. Where the evidence is incomplete or unknown, this book tells you so. A complete list of the original sources used to compile this book is included in the Bibliography. If you have been diagnosed with cancer and are looking for treatment information, this is not the book for you; if someone you love has died or suffered from cancer, this the book may provide some clues as to why a loved one may have developed cancer, and it may make you angry.

Organization

This book book is divided into Part One: What's Personal and Part Two: What's Political. There are a variety of behaviors that fall into the category of "What's Personal" (chapters 2 through 7)—personal lifestyle habits that can be modified to help stop cancer before it starts. Then there are the environmental exposures that fall into the category of "What's Political" (chapters 8 through 10). These are exposures to carcinogenic substances that are beyond our personal control today, but definitely within our collective control for the future. Ultimately, this book puts cancer prevention into your control!

CHAPTER ONE

WHAT IS CANCER?

Cancer is the general term for the abnormal growth of cells. When the abnormal cell reproduces, it has the ability to invade or metastasize to other parts of the body. The actual word *cancer* is Latin for "crab." It was, in fact, the crablike appearance of advanced breast tumors that inspired the Roman physician Galen to name cancer. In Greek, *karkinos* originally meant "crab," too, which is how Hippocrates first identified and classified this illness 2,500 years ago.

Cancer was rarely noted in the ancient world, and it is not mentioned at all in the Bible or the *Yellow Emperor's Classic of Internal Medicine*, the ancient medicine book of China. It began to be seen more extensively around the time of the Industrial Revolution. Actually, the cancer cell itself is not dangerous (unlike bacteria or viruses), but its impact on the rest of the organs is. As it spreads into various parts of the body, it interferes with the jobs of regular cells, confuses other organs, and can wreak havoc. It's basically a terrorist cell, hijacking organs and other cells. Cancer cells use the lymph system to get into the bloodstream and then travel throughout the body. These cells love organs that have multiple blood vessels and nutrients, such as bones, lungs, and brains—common areas where cancer spreads.

Cancer cells are classified into four main groups: carcinoma, sarcoma, leukemia, and lymphoma. A *carcinoma* refers to cancerous cells coming from epithelial cells—cells that line various organs. You'll find carcinomas in organs that tend to secrete something (milk, mucus, digestive juices, and so on). Common sites for carcinomas are breasts, lungs, and colons. Carcinomas account for 80 to 90 percent of all human cancers, and are generally slow-growing. There is always a prefix attached to the word *carcinoma* that tells us where the carcinoma is growing, and the kinds of cells that are involved. An adenocarcinoma, for example, is a carcinoma made of glandular cells. When you just see the word *oma* by itself, it means "benign." An adenoma refers to a clump of benign glandular cells; a fibroma refers to a clump of benign fibrous cells, and so on. When the cells are malignant, the word *carcinoma* is attached to the end, as in adenocarcinoma. It gets even more specific. You'll need to know where the adenocarcinoma itself originated. Think of it like this: *carcinoma* used by itself is as descriptive as saying "sweater." Adenocarcinoma is like saying "wool sweater." More specific descriptions can be "lambs wool sweater" or "angora sweater." And there can be other cancer related prefixes that are similar to saying "blue angora sweater." There are literally hundreds of carcinomas, all described by a different combination of prefixes identifying the parts of the bodies that are involved, the shape of the carcinomas, and so forth.

Sarcomas are cancerous cells coming from supporting connective tissue. Sarcomas are rare and account for only 2 percent of all human cancers but tend to be more aggressive than carcinomas. Again, the prefixes before the word tell you where the sarcoma is located, what it is made of, what shape it has, and so forth, while sometimes sarcomas are named after the doctors who discovered them. The difference between a carcinoma and a sarcoma is equal to the difference between a sweater and a shirt; both are different things, but related. Nonetheless, both have different physical properties, are made of different materials, are available in different colors, and so on. (You can also have a carcinosarcoma—a carcinoma and sarcoma all in one.)

Since cancer cells are living cells, it's in their nature to continue to live. So the first thing cancer cells do is grow. They grow at a faster rate than normal cells. They'll simply begin growing where they first originated, be it in the lung or colon. The second thing cancer cells do is change. Then, they mutate from the other cells that surround them. After they get to a certain age, they want to move out and leave their original nest. So they spread out into surrounding fat and tissue.

A very crucial motive of the cancer cell is to eat. So the cancer cell sends out protein messengers (called *tumor angiogenesis factors*) that create new blood vessels to feed it. If a cancer cell can manage to grow, spread, and eat, it will live and we'll experience this development in the form of a tumor. If any of these functions is stopped, the cancer will die. As you've guessed by now, treatments therefore attempt to stop the cells from growing, stop the cells from changing or mutating, stop the cells from spreading, or stop the cells from eating.

If the cancer continues to live, it will simply continue these same basic behaviors: it will grow bigger; change, and mutate even more, to trick the immune system; and spread out even more by bursting into surrounding structures and into the blood vessels. Finally, if the cells reach adulthood, they'll want to settle down and find a good home, preferably an organ rich in blood vessels, such as the liver, the lungs, or bones. So the cells attach to these blood vessels, and pass through them into such an organ. And they will continue to make themselves comfortable so they can reproduce more and more. This means setting themselves up with a new blood supply to make the organ more conducive to their growth. And so it goes, until the cancer occupies every space in the body. The most important thing to remember is that none of this happens immediately; it can take years for these cancer cells to really spread.

In Situ vs. Invasive

Regardless of whether the cancer is a carcinoma or sarcoma of some kind, the most important words are *in situ* and *invasive*. *In situ* means "in one place." A carcinoma in situ means that the carcinoma is confined to a specific area and has not spread. This is good news and means that the cancer is, by definition, noninvasive and is in an early stage. *Invasive* carcinoma means that the cancer has spread to local tissue, surrounding tissue, lymph nodes, or other organs. This is not good news and means that the cancer is in a later stage. However, even though a cancer may be invasive and in a later stage, it can still be quite treatable.

Differentiated vs. Undifferentiated

Cancer cells are classified into two behavioral categories, *differentiated* and *undifferentiated*. These terms refer to the degree of maturation of the cancer cells or the sophistication of the cancer cells. Differentiated cancer cells resemble the more normal cells of their origin. A differentiated cancer cell that originates in the colon, for example, would look and act like a normal colon cell. In fact, these cancer cells do not reproduce as rapidly as undifferentiated cells. Differentiated cancer cells look different under a microscope from undifferentiated cancer cells. They also have structural differences that allow doctors to tell the type of cancer cell, and therefore predict how rapidly the cell is growing and the degree of malignancy. Both differentiated and undifferentiated cells are often treatable, but key factors are tumor size and lymph node status. Often, you won't find a purely differentiated cell. It may look just moderately abnormal. Because of this, there are subclassifications: moderately differentiated, well-differentiated, or poorly differentiated. These classifications are known as the cell's *grading*.

A high grade means that the cell is immature, poorly differentiated, and therefore faster growing. A low-grade cancer cell is mature, looks more normal or well-differentiated, and is less aggressive. However, this is a terribly basic explanation of cell grading, something that is based on far more complex criteria.

Undifferentiated cancer is made up of very primitive cells that look wild and untamed, bearing little or no resemblance to the cells of origin. This situation is more dangerous because the cells may then spread faster. There are cases, though, when undifferentiated cancer is not very aggressive, despite the fact that it involves more primitive cells. In these cases, the cancer looks wilder than it behaves. This is often the case in breast cancers.

There are also mixes of these different cells, which affect the aggressiveness of the disease. For example, there can be mostly differentiated cells mixed in with a few undifferentiated cells, or vice versa. Whatever is most aggressive will affect the behavior of the cancer. The mostly differentiated cells will slow down whatever undifferentiated cells exist, wheras mostly undifferentiated cells will speed up whatever differentiated cells exist.

HOW CAN YOU STOP CANCER BEFORE IT STARTS?

The recipe for preventing cancer before it begins on the personal front is remembering this holy trinity:

1. *Health enhancement.* This entails doing as many good things for your health as you can, such as eating well and staying physically active, as well as practicing proper hygiene and safe sex. It also means staying mentally and spiritually fit to reduce stress, which is linked to many chronic diseases. Selecting healthy produce and healthy products is another way to enhance health. This also includes choosing products healthy for the environment.

2. *Risk avoidance.* This means avoiding bad things, or *known carcinogens*, such as tobacco (yes, boring old news that doesn't go away), sunburns or UV damage, low-nutrient foods such as junk foods, as well as eliminating as many chemicals as you can from daily use. Switching to personal hygiene products that have fewer industrial chemicals, or using cleaning

products that have fewer industrial chemicals, are easy ways to reduce the risk of exposure to potential carcinogens. It also means finding out about local environmental conditions in your workplace or community and avoiding clear hazards where you can. Learn if your tap water is clean, for example, and if it is not, use an alternative drinking water source or purifier.

3. *Risk reduction.* This means *lowering your exposure* to something you can't help being exposed to, such as occupational toxins, by wearing protective masks or clothing in certain areas (recall the 9/11 health issues), choosing organic produce over pesticide-laden produce, and/or choosing clean water over contaminated water.

We're all born with a big "basement light switch" that is wired for potential diseases, including certain cancers. At birth, most of these switches are off. As we age and develop certain behaviors or live and work in certain environments, these switches can be turned on. It's still unclear which of these switches are being turned on at certain points. All we can do is try to eliminate the triggers that can change our switches from off to on. Any cancer that is linked to the following can be prevented, or stopped before it starts through *lifestyle modification* that involves a combination of health enhancement, risk avoidance, or risk reduction tactics, which include:

- Smoking, substance or alcohol abuse (chapters 2 and 3)
- Poor, high-fat, low-nutrient diets (chapter 3)
- Heavy use of home and personal products made with industrial substances or chemicals (chapter 4)
- Sedentary or inactive lifestyles (chapter 4)
- Exposure to sun damage (chapter 5)

SUMMARY OF RISK FACTORS

In order to practice health enhancement, risk avoidance, or risk reduction, you need to understand what is really meant by the term *risk factors*. What does it mean when you're told you're "at risk" for a particular cancer—or any other disease? It can mean a few different things, depending on the adjective that precedes the word *risk*. When trying to understand risk factors, having a degree in actuarial science really helps. That's because there is a world of difference among absolute, cumulative, relative, modifiable, and attributable risk. *Absolute risk* means that the cancer rate is counted in numbers of cases occurring within a group of people. When you hear, for example, that in the town of Anywhere, "50 out of 100,000 people died last year of a particular cancer," this is absolute risk. The official definition of absolute risk is "the observed or calculated probability of an event in a population under study." So this can be a hypothetical or real population; it's just not relative to any other population. *Cumulative risk* just means "added up." It's a risk per unit of time added up over X units of time, such as a lifetime or a given time frame that a study ran, such as two years or ten years. It can be an estimate or the experiences of a real group of people—but it will be an average of the experiences of that group. So when you read about cumulative risk factors, it is a "guess" of risk based on a number of factors that may include mortalities from a particular cancer in a given area or age group and mortalities of people who share your same medical history. So cumulative risk is not based on you, personally, but on estimates. It's like betting in a horse race. You look at the ages of the horses, the histories, the breeding, the jockeys, and where the race is being run, and you come up with odds. When you read, for example, that "one in eight people over a lifetime" will get a particular cancer, this is a cumulative risk—an average, not an absolute. The problem with a statement like this one is that it tends to underestimate risk in some groups, while over-estimating risk in others.

Then there is *relative risk*, which is based on comparing two populations. For example, when people who eat large amounts of fat are at greater risk for certain cancers than people who have low-fat diets, this refers to relative risk. It directly compares a population that has one type of risk factor with a population that has a different risk factor. It basically compares risk in situation A with risk in situation B (which is usually a standard or constant, such as "no risk factor").

But this doesn't mean that people who eat large amounts of fat cannot alter their diets, or people who smoke cannot quit smoking. When you speak of risk that can be reduced, prevented, or altered through behavior (like quitting smoking or dieting), you're now talking about *modifiable risk* because it is under voluntary control. This is different from a risk marker, such as family history, which cannot be modified. It is also different from *attributable risk*, which refers to a component of one's risk attributable to either a modifiable risk factor, such as diet, or a risk marker, such as family history.

Not all cancers can be linked to an absolute cause, either. For example, breast cancer is not like lung cancer. With lung cancer, we know that at least 70 percent of those who develop it smoke. Therefore, you can absolutely say that smoking causes lung cancer, a cancer that kills more people each year than any other cancer. You can't name one main cause of breast cancer, however. All you can do is count up the people who are diagnosed with the disease, examine the kinds of lifestyles, workplaces, or family histories they have that may be different from those of people without breast cancer, and analyze the effects of each type of difference.

What most of us have been bombarded with since the 1970s are the reports of known risk factors for certain cancers. It's important to understand that many of the "known" risks are conflicting and often controversial. Although one study suggests that this or that increases your risk of some cancers, another study may suggest the contrary. For example, if the odds are less than one in twenty of something being found by chance, it's said to be "statistically significant."

For example, a certain characteristic, such as eye color, makes virtually no difference to anybody's chance of getting a particular cancer. Yet for every twenty studies or comparisons done on this characteristic, one of those studies might show a "significant" departure from the conclusion of "no difference" among cases of people with a particular cancer and the control group (people without that particular cancer). When you see the phrase "statistically significant," remember that it may mean, "We found this purely by chance," even though there may be media hype.

No single risk factor, such as age or diet, can be interpreted as an absolute cause of most cancers. As mentioned earlier, there are many lifestyle changes you can make to significantly lower your risks. In addition, understanding the environmental impact on many cancers will help you put these risks in perspective.

Another final distinction is the difference between association and causation. When you see a statement such as, "Men with prostate cancer were found to eat more fat than men without prostate cancer," this is association. It does not mean that dietary fat causes prostate cancer. When you see the sentence, "Smoking causes lung cancer," this is an example of causation.

The following is an alphabetical list of common, known risk factors for various cancers. The risk factors you can change (avoid or reduce) have an asterisk by the heading.

Age

The risk of many cancers is largely age related because so much cancer is dependent on our behaviors (diet, activity, etc.). The tendency is for most cancers to strike over age 45. When young adults or children develop cancer, it is usually due to exposure to a carcinogen or toxin; in rare cases, there are inherited cancers that strike people at young ages.

Bad Habits*

Any lifestyle indulgence that has proven risk factors is, for the purpose of this book, considered a bad habit. If you smoke, drink an excessive amount of alcohol, or abuse illegal drugs, your risk of getting some diseases is higher than it is for people who don't do these things.

Geography

Who gets cancer depends largely on where people live. Many cancers are "regional." For example, industrialized countries have much higher rates of certain cancers than do underdeveloped countries. Regions dramatically affect the rates of many cancers, and we just don't know why, although economic disparities in access to health care play a role, too. People emigrating from regions with low rates of certain cancers increase their risk when they enter a country with higher incidences of those cancers, which suggests that many cancers are largely caused by environmental factors, such as lifestyle, culture, diet, water, and air quality.

Diet*

As discussed in chapter 3, diet plays an enormous role in cancer risk, and the latest consensus reports are building even stronger evidence for the links between diet and cancer.

Environmental Factors

Environmental factors are extremely important when assessing your risk of cancer, as discussed in chapters 7 through 10.

Estrogen

High levels of estrogen appear to be markers for an increased risk of reproductive cancers, such as breast cancer and endometrial cancer. Sources of extra estrogen include:

- Exposure to DES (diethylstilbestrol), a drug administered to pregnant women from the 1940s to the 1970s to supposedly stop miscarriage. DES daughters are at risk for a variety of reproductive cancers, mainly vaginal and cervical.
- Birth control pills
- Fertility drugs
- Hormone therapy (HT), used to treat the symptoms of menopause and estrogen loss, a risk that has been confirmed with data from the halted Women's Health Initiative Trial, a large multicenter trial, which was stopped in 2002. So-called bioidentical hormones are presumed at this time to carry the same risks, and the phrase "bioidentical hormones" is a marketing term, and not a medical term.
- Body fat. (This is not an external source of estrogen, but it contributes to estrogen production in the body.)
- Environmental estrogens (see chapter 8)
- Hormone-fed meat

Exercise Habits*

Sedentary living breeds ill health and is associated with much higher rates of many cancers, as discussed in chapter 4. The evidence for this link is growing stronger, not weaker.

Family History

As discussed in chapter 6, we are all vulnerable to some diseases more than we are to others.

Education, Income, and Cancer Risk

Not all of us have access to the kind of information or the kind of services we need to stay healthy. Some of this inequality is based on income; some is based on education, literacy, and math literacy (also known as numeracy); some of this is based on healthcare systems. Studies that review socio-economic determinants always find the same thing. The poorer the population, the more disease. Seniors living on fixed incomes, or other economically disadvantaged populations, often do not have access to the right information to stay healthy.

It's been demonstrated time and time again that low-income individuals do not enjoy the same quality of health as their more fortunate neighbors. For example, a study linking life expectancy to neighborhood income found that men living in the wealthiest districts lived an average of 5.7 years longer than men from the poorest neighborhoods, while the average lifespan for women from the richest neighborhoods was almost 2 years longer than that of their low-income counterparts. All of the factors discussed in part 1 of this book, such as good diet with access to nutritious foods, as well as physical activity, are also rich versus poor issues. The rich can afford better food than the poor; the rich have more leisure time than the poor.

In chapter 8, you'll read about occupational hazards. There again, you'll see that occupational cancers are more prevalent among blue-collar workers and nonunionized laborers. We also know that contaminated areas in North America are often inhabited by those with low incomes. Quite simply, many can't afford to leave areas that have become contaminated, while poorer communities tend to be the ones that are home to contaminated waste, landfills, and so on.

Poor nutrition, occupational hazards, lack of access to good screening tests or healthcare counseling, stress associated with being poor (this is not insignificant, by the way), "self-medicating" through addictions such as smoking and alcohol consumption, all play a role in cancer incidence. This may be one reason cancer hits harder in low-income neighborhoods.

Evidence shows that specific cancers reveal considerable differences in the incidence and mortality rates of the rich and the poor. Low socioeconomic status is associated with higher incidence of, and mortality from, the following:

- Stomach cancer
- Lung cancer in men
- Cervical cancer
- Cancers of the mouth, pharynx, larynx, and esophagus

Higher-income groups don't get away scot-free, because there are certain cancers that are linked to "luxury" or "opportunity." These cancers are influenced by higher-fat diets, less physical activity (more cars), and more vacations in the sun. High socio-economic status is associated with a higher incidence of, and mortality from, the following:

- Skin cancer
- Breast cancer
- Prostate cancer
- Colon cancer

As you look at this list, it's easy to see how lifestyle habits affect certain groups. Looking at the "wealthy" cancers: colon, breast, and prostate cancers are associated with too much fat (often because of privileged diets), too much driving, and not enough physical activity. Skin cancer is associated with vacations and leisure time in the sun. So, when it comes to tracking the incidence of disease, it's important to remember that socio-economic differences often bring with them corresponding differences in health-related behaviors, such as smoking, alcohol consumption, and eating habits. Reducing the much-higher rates of smoking among economically disadvantaged groups is perhaps our biggest task in bringing about a reduction in socio-economic inequities in health status. All lifestyle behaviors have to be looked at in the context of the social, economic, environmental, and even political factors (e.g., absence of green space in poorer, urban communities) that motivate them, and that act, in many cases, as barriers to the maintenance of good health.

As stated throughout this book, cancer is caused by many different things, which probably converge. But there are clearly certain carcinogens that cause certain cancers, such as tobacco, which causes most lung cancers. We also know that enhancing our health through nutritious food and regular exercise is definitely associated with lower rates of many cancers. Lean bodies provide less fat in which fat-soluble carcinogens can live, while high-fiber diets and exercise are essential for colon health.

PART ONE

WHAT'S PERSONAL

The information in this section of the book addresses how we can alter our lifestyle, home, or work environment largely to prevent cancer.

CHAPTER 2

TOBACCO WARS

It's not news that smoking causes cancer or that it remains the leading cause of cancer death. What is news is that we are finally seeing rates of lung cancer incidence decline, which is directly related to anti-smoking legislation passed in the last 10 years according to the latest U.S. Centers for Disease Control (CDC) data. Firsthand smoking is by far the leading cause of lung cancers and is a risk factor in a host of other cancers. Smoking accounts for roughly 90 percent of lung cancer cases in men, and 75 to 85 percent of cases in women in the United States and the European Union. One in six premature deaths can be attributed to tobacco use. According to the American Cancer Society, lung cancer continues to be the leading cause of cancer deaths among North American women; in men lung cancer is ahead of prostate cancer as the leading cause of cancer deaths (www.cancer.org).

Lung cancer is uncommon in nonsmokers, but it does occur. Causes of lung cancer in nonsmokers are linked to secondhand smoke exposure (environmental tobacco smoke), radon (see chapter 7), asbestos (see chapter 7), and inhaled chemicals or minerals such as arsenic, nickel, polycyclic aromatic hydrocarbons, or haloethers—exposures you cannot easily control (see chapter 7). But by not smoking, and by reducing your exposure to secondhand smoke (SHS), you can stop *most* lung cancer at the source.

Our children's rights to a healthy environment are being violated by the continued advertising and sale of tobacco. Teens who begin smoking, and grow into tobacco and nicotine-addicted adults, are at high risk of premature death, directly caused by tobacco. And babies and children suffer the effects of secondhand smoke through respiratory disorders and ear infections. Moreover, the number of people who die in fires each year caused by burning cigarettes is not insignificant.

Countless national and international groups have reviewed the effects of tobacco smoke on health, and the evidence has been in for a long time: smoking tobacco causes cancer in smokers, and exposure to secondhand tobacco smoke causes cancer in nonsmokers.

Although the number of smokers in North America has declined substantially over the past twenty-five years, there is still a long way to go.

Studies on tobacco continue to point to the prevalence of smoking among preteens. In fact, more preteens are smoking today than they did in the 1970s. Roughly 23 percent of Americans—adults, children, and adolescents—continue to smoke and use tobacco. The Canadian Lung Association reports that roughly 20 percent of Canadian teens age 12 to 19 smoke daily or occasionally. Tobacco smoke is the most easily removable cancer-causing agent from our environment. Thus, cancer from smoking remains the most preventable form of cancer and premature mortality. According to the American Cancer Society, stopping the use of tobacco could nearly "wipe out lung cancer." The current death toll from lung cancer in the United States is 160,000 deaths annually.

Although there are government initiatives in place to ban smoking from more public places and workplaces throughout North America, there is still not enough support from the public. A 2008 report conducted by the World Health Organization (WHO) acknowledged that while progress has been made, not a single country fully implements all key tobacco control measures. The report presents the first comprehensive analysis of global tobacco use and control efforts, based on data from 179 countries.

Between 1998 and 2004, there have been some encouraging changes, however. Back in 1998, Maryland was the only state to ban smoking in private-sector worksites. In 2004, that number had risen to seven states. As for banning smoking in restaurants in the United States, in 1998, only two states were able to get such legislation passed, and in 2004, the full ban had been implemented in eight states. As of 2012, 81.1% of the U.S. population lives under a smoking ban workplaces, and/or restaurants, and/or bars, by either a state, commonwealth, or local law. And that's why we've seen a drop in lung cancer incidence.

A host of other cancers are caused by smoking. Smokers have a higher risk of developing cancers of the breast, lip, mouth, pharynx, esophagus, bladder, kidneys, and pancreas. Smoking has also been linked to an increased risk of cervical cancer. New research points to higher rates of breast cancer among premenopausal nonsmoking women who have been exposed to secondhand smoke. And users of smokeless tobacco products, such as chewing tobacco and snuff, have a higher risk of developing cancers of the mouth.

Many cancer deaths will occur in former smokers. Quitting smoking does decrease the odds of getting cancer, but former smokers will always be at higher risk than those who have never smoked. The best way to prevent smoking-associated cancer deaths is never to smoke. And for smokers, the earlier you quit, the greater the benefit.

Carcinogens in Tobacco

In 1989, the U.S. Surgeon General released a report listing forty-three carcinogenic agents found in tobacco smoke, as classified by the International Agency for Research on Cancer (IARC). This report continues to be renewed, and the full monographs are available under the search "tobacco" at http://monographs.iarc.fr

SECONDHAND TOBACCO SMOKE

What should really spark some action concerning tobacco and smoking is that nonsmokers are vulnerable to tobacco-related cancers. Secondhand smoke (SHS), is recognized as a leading cause of heart disease and lung cancer in nonsmokers, sudden infant death syndrome, (SIDS) in infants, and respiratory problems in children and adults. The 1986 report of the U.S. Surgeon General concluded that involuntary exposure to secondhand smoke could cause tobacco-related diseases, including lung cancer. This landmark document proved that no one is without risk, and changed the focus of a decision not to smoke from a lifestyle issue to an environmental health hazard.

In 1996, a report from the U.S. Environmental Protection Agency (EPA) confirmed the Surgeon General's conclusions by classifying SHS as a Class A carcinogen, the most incriminating category of cancer-causing agents. The report found that SHS, which is a combination of sidestream and exhaled smoke, causes lung cancer in nonsmokers and impairs the health of infants and children. To help make all North American public areas smoke-free, we need to support government initiatives rather than fight them. Bold steps toward protecting children from secondhand smoke are laws that ban smoking in vehicles with children. The first such law was passed in Canada in 2007; now several U.S. states have passed laws that make it illegal to smoke in a vehicle with anyone under the age of 18 inside.

Lung Cancer in Never Smokers

A number of recent studies and reveiws noted that 15 percent of men and 53 percent of women with lung cancer worldwide are "never smokers." Lung cancer in never smokers (LCINS) disproportionately affects women more than men. The most current evidence suggests that LCINS is a distinct disease entity with unique molecular and biological characteristics. Some of the factors that could explain the occurrence of LCINS are, as noted in this review, secondhand smoke, exposure to cooking fumes inherited genetic susceptibility, occupational and environmental exposure, hormonal factors, pre-existing lung disease, and oncogenic viruses, such as human papillomavirus. The research into LCINS is ongoing as of this writing.

Pregnancy and Infants

Fetuses and children whose parents smoke are the most vulnerable to exposure. Respiratory illnesses are more common in children born to smokers, while smoking during pregnancy can lead to the premature rupture of membranes, premature birth, perinatal death, placental abnormalities, and bleeding during pregnancy.

Breastfeeding mothers who smoke will find that their milk supply is affected by nicotine, so that they may make less milk. As a result, they may be depriving their children of the benefits of breastfeeding, and exposing them to the dangers of formula feeding (such as numerous gastrointestinal problems). The American Academy of Pediatrics (AAP) lists any amount of nicotine as contraindicated during breastfeeding. Too much nicotine can cause shock, vomiting, diarrhea, rapid heart rate, and restlessness in the baby. Recent research suggests that a baby's sleep patterns can be greatly affected by nicotine. A study from the journal *Pediatrics* in 2007 notes that babies who are breastfed by smoking mothers spend less time in active sleep in the short term. Evidently, as greater doses of nicotine are delivered, the infants spent less time in active sleep. Secondhand smoke is, arguably, even more damaging to your baby than nicotine levels in breast milk. There are dozens of studies that conclude babies who breathe in smoke from one or both parents simply do not feel as well as the babies born to nonsmokers. Secondhand smoke can also cause pneumonia, bronchitis or even sudden infant death syndrome. The American Academy of Pediatrics notes on its Web site (as of 2008), that nearly 40 percent of U.S. children are exposed to SHS and "if current tobacco use patterns persist, an estimated 6.4 million children will die prematurely from a smoking-related disease."

WAGING WAR ON TOBACCO

The war on tobacco will be won only with individual and community support. Through education, counseling, school and workplace programs, and some antismoking legislation, we can have a large impact and help people avoid the effects of tobacco smoke. The goal of antitobacco programs is simple: to deter young people from smoking, to encourage smokers to quit, and to protect the public from health risks associated with secondhand smoke.

Raising Tobacco Taxes

If you'd like to see a reduction in smoking, write to your local or federal government and demand that taxes on tobacco be raised to the maximum amount. There is strong evidence to suggest that people smoke less when they are forced to pay more for their addiction.

Restricting Access to Tobacco Products

Although a minimum age for the purchase of tobacco has been in place for at least a decade in most states and provinces, efforts to enforce these restrictions are usually weak. By imposing fines on retailers who sell cigarettes to minors, and by initiating education programs to make retailers aware of the penalties, as well as the role they can play in preventing teens from smoking in the first place, fewer retailers will continue to sell tobacco to minors, and their access to cigarettes will be further restricted. Cigarettes should not be made available everywhere. But in many regions in North America, they are. Each state or province could establish a Tobacco Control Board or agency to assume responsibility for the control of tobacco products and coordinate efforts to limit their availability. In more recent years, partnerships of public health agencies, school boards, and retailers are beginning to form coalitions to actively stop the flow of tobacco products to youth. As one of its highest priorities such an agency might also have the right to investigate the practices of the tobacco industry. The job of a regulatory commission or board would be to:

- Recommend new public policy and report directly to the Department of Health and Human Services in the United States or to Health Canada

31

- License or control access to tobacco products
- Regulate promotional activities of the tobacco industry
- Enforce cost-recovery methods of smoking-related health costs
- Work with other organizations to develop information and educational strategies
- Assist health professionals and institutions in counseling smokers about methods of quitting by instituting pay-by-performance bonuses. In the United Kingdom, for example, physicians get paid more if their patients actually quit smoking due to their counseling efforts
- Control the export of tobacco products

Designation of Tobacco as a Hazardous Product

You may have seen some of these product-label warnings: Smoking Causes Lung Cancer; Smoking during Pregnancy Can Harm Your Baby; Smoking May Cause Heart Disease. Ideally, tobacco should be designated a hazardous product under the appropriate laws in the United States and Canada. Designating tobacco as a hazardous product would really help legislators pass the kinds of laws that can restrict smoking and cut down its appeal. This designation would allow plain packaging, enlarge package warnings, and allow tobacco to be taxed at the earlier points of production and manufacture. In 2012, the first country to affix graphic pictures of tobacco-related cancers was Australia. The High Court in Australia ruled that cigarette manufacturers' names will be published in a small generic font, and large graphic health warnings will dominate the package, along with disturbing, graphic visuals.

Banning Tobacco Advertising and Sponsorship

Why do we still see advertisements for tobacco in popular magazines (particularly, women's magazines)? Tobacco companies should not be allowed to sponsor sports or cultural events, or other public activities. It is even suspect for tobacco companies to sponsor "antismoking" campaigns using their logos. Any "good" that tobacco companies do sends subliminal messages to the public—particularly to women, children, and teenagers—that cigarettes are somehow linked to something acceptable.

Although there have been strong efforts by North American governments to limit cigarette advertising, we still see lively, colorful print advertisements in magazines and on billboards that promote smoking. Any kind of advertising, including sponsorship, allows tobacco companies to sport their logos. Some progress is being made but the tobacco companies pour billions of dollars into point of purchase advertising and promotional items (e.g., cell phone charms inside cigarette packs and discount cigarette coupons) to market their products.

Print advertising in women's magazines continues to send seductive messages to young women, who link smoking to beauty and, most of all, to thinness. As a consumer, you have the power to stop this by boycotting events that are sponsored by tobacco companies and then by contacting the boycotted organization to say that it has lost you as a patron because of its willingness to use tobacco dollars. Tobacco sponsorship is unethical in all but one scenario: paying for or sponsoring the treatment of smoking-related illnesses and compensating people who are debilitated by smoking-related illnesses.

Restricting or prohibiting sponsorship may appear to punish the organizations that need the money, but we cannot afford to continue to send mixed messages. Public health and primary prevention experts suggest that governments prohibit the use of tobacco product names, trademarks, colors, and logos in all tobacco-sponsorship advertising. Health Canada's Tobacco Act, in 2003, stipulated that "it is against the law to promote sponsorship by putting the name of a tobacco company or its product-related brand elements on a permanent sports or cultural facility, such as an arena or theatre."

Removing the incentive for organizations to accept sponsorship from the tobacco industry is another way to address the problem. The state of Victoria, Australia, for example, formed the Victoria Health Promotion Foundation with just such an incentive in mind. Funded by tobacco taxes, the foundation's mandate is to support the sports and cultural groups that refuse tobacco industry funding. Other governments could offer a similar program by working with cancer and other health organizations to pool resources to provide such support, especially by using some of the revenue from tobacco taxation. And if we increase taxes on tobacco even further, the eventual return could be funneled back into the healthcare system, thereby improving the quality of life for everyone.

Making Good Use of Tobacco Dollars

Billions per year are spent treating people with smoking-related illnesses. This is an enormous economic burden to place on a society, especially when it is clear that *primary prevention is possible*. Most U.S. states have launched lawsuits against the tobacco industry. In 1998, following the publication of the *Vanity Fair* article titled "The Man Who Knew Too Much," lawsuits against big tobacco, filed first by Mississippi, and then by forty other states, were eventually settled at US$246 billion. Unfortunately, many states do not use these funds for comprehensive tobacco control programs. Other jurisdictions have considered increased taxation on the tobacco industry as a means of seeking payback for the harm caused by the sale of its products. However, many states do not earmark tobacco tax revenues for tobacco control programs; rather, they often use the revenues to balance the budget.

Investigating Tobacco

The 1999 film *The Insider* documents the ugly truth about what the tobacco industry has suppressed. Since 1996, investigations and lawsuits into harmful and clearly unethical tobacco industry practices revealed shocking information that showed companies:

- Suppressing evidence linking tobacco with ill health
- Using nicotine to enhance the addictive properties of tobacco In this case, cigarette manufacturing's is "nicotine delivery"
- Circulating misleading information, masking the health consequences of smoking
- Using advertising that targets vulnerable groups. These advertising campaigns sink to terrible lows in their intent to appeal to children, young women, and low-income individuals
- Exporting tobacco products to developing nations, often with accompanying advertising aimed at minors or other groups who don't have the income to support their nicotine addiction

Counseling against Smoking

Healthcare providers are bound by professional ethics and their legal duties of care to counsel you and your family against harmful practices that can affect your health. That includes counseling against smoking and SHS. The advice and support of a physician really can help a smoker to quit, or can even prevent someone from starting. Unfortunately, not all healthcare providers adequately counsel their patients about the dangers of smoking or exposure to SHS.

Healthcare providers include all health professionals, such as nurses, pharmacists, nurse practitioners, dentists, dermatologists, and community health workers. Counseling on all these levels can help in the war against tobacco. Every state has a free telephone hotline available to help tobacco users quit: 1-800-QUIT-NOW.

WOMEN AND SMOKING

The results are in: many young women begin smoking to control their weight. Roughly 60 percent of women in the United States are actually overweight, according to the CDC; 75 percent of North American women believe they are overweight, even when their body weight is normal for their size, height, and age.

Tobacco advertisements in women's magazines continue to sell the message to young women that smoking is beautiful or glamorous. Boycotting women's magazines or other women's events that accept tobacco advertising is one thing you, as a consumer, can do with follow-up letters to the organizations explaining your reasons, is an important act of protest you, as a consumer, have the power to make.

Smoking and Weight Control

Many women use cigarettes as a tool for weight loss, or worse, revisit the habit long after they've quit if they are dieting. Smoking suppresses the appetite and satisfies mouth hunger—the need to have something in your mouth. But the irony is that smoking and obesity often coexist. Although some women begin to smoke in their teens as a way to lose weight, studies show that this approach doesn't work. Smoking teens are just as likely to become obese over time as are nonsmoking teens. Ironically, it was found that the more a person weighed, the more cigarettes she smoked. In the long run, smokers often wound up weighing more than nonsmokers because they substituted food for nicotine when they quit or attempted to quit.

35

This leads not only to higher rates of smoking-related cancers but also a host of health problems linked to the catastrophic quartet of obesity, smoking, sedentary, lifestyle, high blood pressure, and/or high cholesterol. Smoking women also tend to go into earlier menopause, while older smokers have 20 to 30 percent less bone mass than nonsmokers, predisposing them to bone loss and osteoporosis-linked fractures.

Cooking Oil Smoke: Cause for Lung Cancer?

In the late 1990s, it was discovered that Chinese women world-wide were developing lung cancer in high numbers, yet few of them smoked. The lung cancers were linked to oil smoke from wok cooking. The first study linking cooking fume exposure and lung cancer among Chinese females using a quantitative approach, one of the gold standards in evidence-based research, was published by Chinese investigators in 2006 in the journal *Cancer Research*. The investigators looked at the "association between lung cancer and fumes emitted from Chinese-style cooking among Hong Kong Chinese women using a composite index for lifetime cumulative exposure and taking into account the influence of various potential confounding factors." They concluded that "there was strong evidence that cumulative exposure to cooking by means of any form of frying could increase the risk of lung cancer in Hong Kong nonsmoking women."

A CIGAR IS NOT JUST A CIGAR

Cigar smoking came back into vogue in the late 1990s, and the popularity of cigars with youth, according to the American Lung Association, is staggering. By 2005, 14.9 percent of high school students were current cigar smokers. According to the State Tobacco Activity Tracking Estimates by the CDC, in over 6 percent of U.S. adults are cigar users. Ninety percent of the total are men. An estimated 6 million U.S. teenagers (26.7 percent) age 14 to19—4.3 million males (37 percent) and 1.7 million females (16 percent)—smoked at least one cigar within the past year. U.S. students in grades 9 to 12 who smoked cigarettes or used smokeless tobacco products also were more likely to report smoking cigars. Nearly three-fourths of male and one-third of female cigarette and smokeless tobacco users reported smoking at least one cigar in the past year, according to the CDC.

When you smoke a cigar, you're getting filler, binder, and wrapper, which are made of air-cured and fermented tobaccos. Like cigarette tobacco, lit cigars emit more than 4,000 chemicals, of which 43 are known to cause cancer. The SHS emitted from a cigar is more deadly than the tobacco smoke from cigarettes.

Since cigars are not inhaled and are expensive, few people are addicted, and people tend to smoke them as a pastime rather than as an all-the-time event. Cigar smoking is a dangerous activity nonetheless, and it is still a cause of mouth and other cancers. Cigar and pipe smoking have the same adverse effects on periodontal health and tooth loss as cigarette smoking. Cigar (and pipe) smokers have higher death rates than nonsmokers for most smoking-related diseases, although they are not nearly as high as death rates in cigarette smokers. When the nicotine is absorbed through the mouth, however, cigar/pipe smokers, as well as anyone using chewing tobacco or snuff, are at higher risk of laryngeal, oral, and esophageal cancers.

Cigar/pipe smokers also have higher death rates than nonsmokers from chronic obstructive lung disease as well as from lung cancer. Cigar smoking is a pastime that is being sold to women as something that is attractive and sexy. And women are buying into it, when in fact they are much more attracted to the maleness of the cigar and the "male world" it evokes for them. It is vital to start anticigar smoking campaigns to end mouth and other related cancers. Since this trend is attractive to higher-income groups, anticigar smoking campaigns should be targeting universities and other centers of higher learning, as well as large corporations.

QUITTING SMOKING

In order to prevent smoking-related lung cancer, which accounts for roughly 90 percent of lung cancers—still the top killer cancer—and other smoking-related diseases, we can't just focus on getting people to quit smoking; we have to focus on preventing people from starting. Studies show that any real health benefits that long-term ex-smokers (that is, people who smoked from their teen years until age 55 or so) gain from quitting are not noticeable until at least fifteen years after they quit. This fact was shown in the American Cancer Society's Cancer Prevention Study, where the death rates of former smokers did not begin to match those of never-smokers until fifteen to twenty years after the smokers quit. If you smoked for only a short period of time, or quit smoking in your thirties or forties, the health benefits will be seen much more quickly. The fact remains that it is never too late to quit.

Tobacco Dependence Treatment

If you are attempting to quit smoking through some of the tobacco treatment methods, request reimbursement from your cigarette-brand manufacturer. You should also seek out other quitters who may want to launch a class action suit for recovering tobacco treatment costs from tobacco manufacturers. And you may want to ask your workplace to fund a tobacco treatment program using local or state funding from government agencies to fund the program. As of this writing, here is a summary of the types of methods people use for quitting smoking:

- *Behavioral counseling.* Behavioral counseling, either group or individual, can raise the rate of abstinence from 20 to 25 percent. This approach to tobacco treatment aims to change the mental processes of smoking, reinforce the benefits of not smoking, and teach skills to help the smoker avoid the urge to smoke.
- *Nicotine replacement.* The FDA has approved five types of nicotine replacement therapy: nicotine gum, patch, inhalers, nasal spray, and lozenges. There are several types of products available, and your doctor or pharmacist can guide you. You can also visit the American Cancer Society Web site at www.cancer.org for further information.
- *Prescription medications.* A variety of prescription drugs have been approved for use in quitting smoking, and these can be prescribed by any primary care physician, who will assess whether they conflict with other medications you may be taking. .
- *Alternative therapies.* Hypnosis, meditation, and acupuncture have helped some smokers quit. In the case of hypnosis and meditation, sessions may be private or part of a group tobacco treatment program.

CHAPTER 3

DIET

This chapter explores what we absolutely know about the role diet plays in cancer incidence, as well as *what we suspect, but can't prove* about diet and cancer. The most comprehensive summary of diet and cancer done to date is a report that came out in November 2007 entitled *Food, Nutrition, Physical Activity, and the Prevention of Cancer: A Global Perspective* available online at www.dietandcancerreport.org. Since the first report came out in 1997, an enormous amount of scientific literature on the topic has been produced, making the need for an update very clear. This report was commissioned by the executive officers of the World Cancer Research Fund (WCRF) and the American Institute for Cancer Research (AICR). It contains the work of many organizations and individual experts, and it was designed to address the primary prevention of cancer from a global perspective. All aspects of food and nutrition likely to reduce or increase cancer risk were reviewed. The panel assembled for the report agreed on a consistent method to assess the various types of scientific evidence. This AICR report was an exhaustive review of the scientific and other expert literature published over the last five years, linking foods, nutrition, food processing, dietary patterns, and related factors with the risk of human cancers worldwide.

This chapter is designed to help you sort out what to take seriously, or lightly, in the news when you hear: "A new study says…"

WHAT YOU EAT AND DRINK

Obesity is strongly associated with several cancers, most notably kidney, endometrial, breast, colon, rectal, and gallbladder cancers. Body fat also increases cancers that are estrogen-dependent because fat cells make estrogen; the estrogen your body produces can make a cancer cell thrive. Estrogen-dependent cancers include breast, endometrial, and colon cancers. Thus, in addition to the other health risks associated with obesity discussed in previous chapters, these cancers can be added to the list.

Obesity aside, human and animal studies point to the same conclusion: diet can both increase your risk of cancer and reduce your risk. Dietary risk factors have been linked to a number of common cancers, including stomach, breast, colon, and prostate. Protective factors, especially those derived from plant foods such as fruits and vegetables, have been associated with a reduced risk of many cancers. Most cancer experts agree that next to smoking, diet is the second-leading modifiable cause of cancer. That means, by modifying your diet, you can reduce your risk of cancer.

What the Studies Show

Overall, studies show that people who consume large amounts of dietary fat and meat are more likely to develop, and die from, breast and colon cancer, as well as cancers of the ovary, kidney, endometrium (lining of the uterus), and lung. One of the problems with many epidemiological studies is that while they indicate trends in particular groups of people, they can't tell us how and why each individual's diet affects him or her. There are many other factors that can affect diet, including childbearing patterns, genetics, activity levels, and stress.

Studies measuring dietary links to cancer are fraught with complications. For example, it's hard for study participants to remember their food intake accurately, even if they are keeping journals. And since there are many components within one item, such as a hamburger (starches, proteins, chemicals in condiments, vegetables on top of the hamburger, and cooking method), even a superb record from a study participant can be hard to analyze.

Just how much cancer is linked to a poor diet? Estimates vary from 15 to 75 percent, but in light of more recent studies, it looks as if we're hovering at 30 percent, which is very significant. That said, based on studies to date, some cancers, such as colon and rectal cancer, can absolutely be linked to diet, while the link between diet and other cancers still remains foggy, such as the link between diet and breast cancer. Here is the best information we have to date.

Food Groups and Cancer

The following is what we know so far about various food groups and cancer risk. The term *convincing evidence* means there is enough evidence to demonstrate an absolute link; the term *probable* refers to a strong link; the term *possible* refers to an established link; the term *insufficient evidence* means a link has been made in the published studies, but there is not enough backup from other studies that clearly demonstrates that the link is serious enough to be considered; the term *no relationship* means just that—there is no study published in the literature showing a link exists, or, a study has revealed that a suspected link is not there.

Carbohydrates

It is possible that fiber can decrease the risk of colon, rectum, pancreatic, and breast cancers. It is also possible that refined starchy diets, which are usually high in salt, can increase the risk of stomach, colon, and rectal cancers. It is possible that whole-grain cereals decrease the risk of stomach cancer, whereas refined cereals can increase the risk of esophageal cancers. There is insufficient evidence, however, to demonstrate that whole-grain cereals can decrease the risk of colon cancer.

Fat

There is no relationship so far between high cholesterol and breast cancer, or of "good fats" (see chapter 3) and breast cancer, either. It is possible, however, that high cholesterol levels can increase the risk of lung cancer and pancreatic cancer, but there is insufficient evidence to demonstrate that cholesterol can increase the risk endometrial cancer.

It is possible that diets high in total fat, which contribute to obesity and body size, can increase the risk of lung, colon, rectum, breast, and prostate cancers. There is insufficient evidence to demonstrate a link between total fat intake and ovarian, endometrial, and bladder cancers. It is possible that diets high in saturated fats can increase the risk of lung, colon, rectum, breast, endometrium, and prostate cancers. There is insufficient evidence to demonstrate a link between saturated fat intake and ovarian cancer.

Vegetables and Fruits

There is convincing evidence that a diet rich in fruits and vegetables decreases the risk of the following cancers: mouth and pharynx, esophageal, lung, stomach, colon, and rectal (vegetables only). There is probable evidence that vegetables and fruits can decrease the risk of larynx, pancreatic, breast, and bladder cancers. There is possible evidence that fruits and vegetables can decrease the risk of the following cancers: cervical, ovarian, endometrial, thyroid, liver (veggies only), prostate (veggies only), and kidney (veggies only). There are few studies done on legumes and cancer risk, but the report notes that dried beans such as red, black, pinto, and navy beans; garbanzos; split peas; and lentils offer a lot of fiber and protein, and are an excellent, daily healthy choice.

Meat, Poultry, Fish, and Eggs

Dietary guidelines recommend generally that you cut back on meat in order to make room for greater portions of vegetables, fruits, whole grains, and beans. They also make the point that red meat is a special case, and that there is convincing evidence that beef, lamb, and pork increase your chances of developing colorectal cancer. An expert panel concluded that a safe amount of lean red meat per week is 18 ounces, and the panel furthermore recommends cutting back on processed meats (sausage, bacon, ham, and lunch meats), since the evidence is convincing that these meats raise your risk of colorectal cancer as well. No evidence connects either fish or poultry consumption to increased cancer risk.

Whole Grains

Adding whole grains, such as brown rice, kasha, bulgur, or quinoa to your diet can be a healthier choice than eating potatoes and white rice. It's advisable that if you have either bread or rolls with a meal, choose a product with whole wheat flour. A recent study in the November 2007 issue of the *American Journal of Epidemiology* cites epidemiological data that support the hypothesis that consuming more whole grain or high-fiber foods may reduce the risk of pancreatic cancer.

Milk and Dairy Products

At this time, the evidence surrounding milk and dairy products and cancer links specifically is very low. The only thing that can be said is that it is possible that too much milk and dairy can increase the risk of prostate and kidney cancer. A December 2007 study in the *American Journal of Clinical Nutrition* notes that a diet rich in dairy products during childhood is associated with a greater risk of colorectal cancer in adulthood. See also Fat, where most of the studies focus on saturated fats, based on animal fats. See also Vitamins; many studies on vitamin D, which is in milk and dairy products have been done.

Minerals from Various Food Groups

Right now, we know it's possible that selenium decreases lung cancer as well as possibly prostate cancer; however, there is insufficient evidence to demonstrate that selenium decreases stomach, liver, or thyroid cancer or that vitamin D decreases colon and rectal cancer. It is probable that not enough iodine increases the risk of thyroid cancer, yet it is possible that too much iodine increases the risk of thyroid cancer. There is insufficient evidence to show that iron increases the risk of liver, colon, or rectal cancers and no relationship between colon cancer and the intake of calcium and selenium.

Vitamins from the Various Food Groups

There's a reason why, in chapters 3 and 4, I reiterate how important it is to have a diet rich in fruits and vegetables. It is because the vitamins in those foods are an important part of decreasing cancer risk. So far, it is probable that carotenoids (which include the plant precursors of vitamin A) decrease the risk of lung cancer, while vitamin C decreases the risk of stomach cancer. It is possible that carotenoids decrease the risk of esophageal, stomach, colon, rectum, breast, and cervical cancers, and that vitamin C decreases the risk of mouth, pharynx, esophageal, lung, pancreatic, and cervical cancers. It is also possible that vitamin E decreases the risk of lung and cervical cancers. There is insufficient evidence to demonstrate, however, that carotenoids can decrease laryngeal, ovarian, endometrial, or bladder cancers; or that vitamin C decreases larynx, colon, rectum, breast, or bladder cancers; that retinol decreases bladder cancer; that vitamin E decreases colon or rectal cancer, or that folate and methionine decrease colon or rectal cancer.

Right now, there is no relationship between vitamin C and prostate cancer; retinol and lung, stomach, breast, or cervical cancers; vitamin E and stomach and breast cancers, or folate and cervical cancer.

Diet and Colon Cancer

Of all the studies done on the link between cancer and dietary fat, the strongest connections can be made between high-fat diets and colon cancer. In other words, people who consume high quantities of fat have higher rates of colon cancer; people who consume low quantities of fat have lower rates of colon cancer.

As for fiber, studies show that people who consume high quantities of fiber have lower rates of colon cancer, whereas people who consume low quantities of fiber have higher rates of colon cancer. The AICR report notes that since the mid-1990s, evidence for a protective effect of dietary fiber (cereals, grains, and other plant foods) has become somewhat stronger. In addition, people who have regular bowel movements have lower incidences of colon cancer than do people who are chronically constipated. It's safe to say that by lowering fat and increasing fiber, you can possibly reduce your risk of colon cancer. In fact, Canadian experts believe that by following a low-fat, high-fiber diet, you may be able to avoid 90 percent of all stomach and colon cancers, and 20 percent of gallbladder, pancreatic, mouth, pharynx, and esophageal cancers.

Diet and Breast Cancer

We know that breast cancer rates are four to seven times higher in North America than in Asia. When Asian women move to North America, their risk doubles over a decade and they seem to acquire breast cancer at North American rates after several generations. We don't know what accounts for this difference. Is it diet—are we eating something we shouldn't or are they eating some foods when in Asia that we should? For example, Japanese diets average roughly 15 percent calories from fat, whereas North American diets average about 40 percent calories from fat. The traditional low-fat Japanese diet of rice, vegetables, and fish is light-years away from the meat and high-fat diet of North Americans.

The Japanese diet is also rich in plant estrogens (called *phytoestrogens*), such as tofu. Phytoestrogens act as weak estrogens, which interfere with ordinary estrogen production. And since estrogen seems to promote breast tumors, anything that interferes with estrogen should, theoretically, cut the risk. Some studies suggest that phytoestrogens may be associated with lower rates of breast cancer and less severe menopausal symptoms. But like most research on cancer prevention, to this date there is conflicting evidence. A 2007 paper in the journal *CA: A Cancer Journal for Clinicians* points out that the data regarding the role of phytoestrogens in breast cancer prevention is conflicting, yet early exposure to phytoestrogens in the diet in childhood and early adolescence may be protective. Phytoestrogens are found in a variety of fruits and vegetables, including all soybean and linseed products, apples, alfalfa sprouts, split peas, and spinach.

Perhaps culture is a large piece in the puzzle. For example, you'll find fewer children, more birth control, and less breastfeeding in the West as opposed to more children, less birth control, and more breastfeeding in Asian cultures. Some even wonder about the effect of more physical activity on cancer risk in Asian women versus in sedentary Western women.

Studies on dietary fat and breast cancer have not been able to absolutely prove that high-fat diets are linked to a greater breast cancer risk, however. A review paper from the journal *Cancer* in June 2007 states, "Among the prospective epidemiological studies conducted on diet and breast cancer incidence and gene-diet interactions and breast cancer incidence, to date there is no association that is consistent, strong, and statistically significant, with the exception of alcohol intake, overweight, and weight gain." The fat and breast cancer issue has polarized breast cancer researchers. Some will tell you that the proof is in the geography: countries with high-fat diets simply have more breast cancer. Others will tell you that there are too many variables geographically and culturally that need to be studied before the fat theory becomes fact.

What you've probably heard most about is the U.S. Nurses' Health Study, where half of the nurses enrolled (who were followed over several years) received 44 percent of their daily calories from fat, while the other half received 23 percent of their daily calories from fat. This study was analyzed by Harvard University's Walter Willett, who concluded that the study showed no difference in breast cancer risk between the two groups. Similar studies on dietary fat found the same results.

Critics of the Nurses' Health Study argue that in order to see a difference, the fat-cutting nurses should have been getting no more than 15 percent of their calories from fat. Other problems with dietary fat studies are that food-frequency questionnaires are used to measure what people are eating, which are pretty crude measurement tools. Researchers also question the timing of dietary fat in a woman's life cycle. Some wonder whether low-fat diets have greater impact on breast cancer risk in childhood and adolescence, when breasts are still forming, than in adulthood, when breasts are mature.

We may know the answers to some of these questions in the year 2010, when the results from the largest dietary fat study to date are due. The Women's Health Initiative is a $628 million health trial involving 164,000 U.S. women. It intends to test whether a low-fat diet that is high in fruits, vegetables, and grains leads to lower breast cancer incidence in postmenopausal women than does the typical Western diet. Among some of the selective findings that the initiative has published to date, including three papers in the *Journal of the American Medical Association* in February 2006, is the finding that reducing total fat intake may have a small effect on risk of breast cancer, but, evidently, no effect on the risk of colorectal cancer.

Finally, researchers published a 1998 report that suggested a 40 percent increased risk of breast cancer in women who consumed higher levels of trans-fatty acids (see chapters 3 and 8). The risk was highest among women who consume low levels of polyunsaturated fats and high levels of trans-fatty acids.

Food, Body Fat, and Environmental Toxins: What We Can't Prove, but Suspect

Some environmental scientists, such as Dr. Sandra Steingraber, author of *Living Downstream: An Ecologist Looks at Cancer and the Environment*, hypothesize that body fat serves as an excellent host for fat-soluble toxins, such as organochlorines, which are discussed more in chapter 8.

The most serious hazards affecting our food are what are called *persistent toxic substances*. These are so named because they are, well, persistent. They remain in the biophysical environment for long periods of time and become widely dispersed, establishing themselves in the plants and animals (including humans!) that ingest them as part of the food chain. Sadly, the ecosystem is incapable of breaking down many of these substances; because they are not naturally occurring chemicals (with their own built-in metabolic pathways for detoxifying themselves), the ecosystem has no way to absorb them. In fact, many of these chemicals have been developed because they are not readily metabolized and detoxified! They stick around and by so doing, cause any number of adverse health effects, including cancer in humans and animals. How environmental toxins and carcinogens enter our food is discussed more in chapter 8.

Dietary Guidelines for Preventing Cancer

1. Reduce intake of saturated fat, which is linked to higher rates of colon, ovarian, and prostate cancers. (Red meat is associated more with colon and advanced prostate cancer.)

2. Daily consumption of fresh fruits and vegetables may reduce the risks of a number of cancers, including those of the mouth, pharynx, esophagus, stomach, colon, rectum, larynx, lung, breast, and bladder.

3. Both soluble and insoluble fiber (see chapter 8) are good for you; experts are not entirely sure why. Is it the beneficial ingredients in high-fiber foods? Is it the regularity that fiber promotes? Right now, since all the good foods are also high in fiber, we are promoting high-fiber diets, but some experts think it's better to promote a high fruit and vegetable diet.

The AICR's Panel specifically suggests the following eight general recommendations, plus two special recommendations:

1. *Body fatness.* Be as lean as possible within the normal range of body weight.

2. *Physical activity.* Be physically active for at least thirty minutes every day.

3. *Foods and drinks that promote weight gain.* Limit consumption of energy-dense foods (particularly processed foods high in sugar, or low in fiber, or high in fat), and avoid sugary drinks.

4. *Plant foods.* Eat foods mostly of plant origin, including vegetables, fruits, whole grains, and legumes.

5. *Animal foods.* Limit intake of red meat, and avoid processed meat.

6. *Alcoholic drinks.* If consumed at all, limit alcoholic drinks to two for men and one for women a day.

7. *Preservation, processing, preparation.* Limit consumption of salty foods and foods processed with salt.

8. *Dietary supplements.* Aim to meet nutritional needs through diet alone.

9. *Breastfeeding.* It's best for mothers to breastfeed exclusively for six months, and then add other liquids and foods.

10. *Cancer survivors.* After treatment, cancer survivors should follow the recommendations for cancer prevention.

What you basically need to understand about good diets versus bad diets is that people who consume less saturated fats and fewer empty calories (high-starch or high-sugar items) and more fiber are generally healthier. A low-fat, high-fiber diet will reduce your risk of colon cancer, and possibly other cancers, and will reduce your risk of heart disease and diabetes.

WHO CAN HELP US EAT BETTER?

Knowing all the fiber, fat, and sugar information is not going to help you eat well if you don't have access to a healthy, high-quality food supply or food labels you can read and understand. So what can we do as consumers to help business and government make it easier for us?

When we think about who protects our diet we may look to departments or ministries of health, food, water, agriculture, finance, education, industry, social services, and trade. Agricultural food departments or ministries are certainly the most important players in our diet, but don't forget that they have to work together with food retailers and food services to help promote high-quality foods, healthy eating habits, and, most important, access to a healthy food supply. By looking at the way food is produced, stored, and distributed, policies can be introduced by government and industry to help ensure that good food is available to all of us.

Getting the Food Industry on Our Side

Ideally, we want those in the food industry responsible for the production of fruit, vegetables, and high-fiber grain products, as well as the producers and distributors of lower-fat meat and dairy products, to get more of their foods on food retailers' shelves. You may have tried to "healthy food-shop" in smaller cities or towns and noticed the absence of fresh foods or the absence of variety in "outside aisles." This is a food industry and food distribution problem. The first thing you can do is contact your local food retailers and ask them where they buy their produce so you can locate the right channels to voice your concerns.

You may also notice that you can buy seven different kinds of brand-name cereals but can't find a bag of natural oats or generic natural grain cereals. Again, this is a food industry problem, whereby brand-name, more expensive, and less nutritious products are often shelved because the profit margins are higher. In these cases, you can contact the food industry and make your demands known for more variety in products, particularly generic alternatives to brand names. Since the food industry is very concerned with what consumers want, they are more apt to respond to consumer demands. Recent wins by individual consumer complaints have resulted in the food industry giving in to our demands. We now have products without trans fats and without high fructose corn syrup—with call-out labels that advertise it as a "plus".

Food Labels

Surveys continuously reveal that shoppers consider nutrition to be either very important or extremely important. They also reveal that consumers rely on packages and labels for nutrition information, but that in most cases, they find the ingredients list of certain products—especially processed and artificial food products—hard to decipher. In cases where food products are designed to mimic or substitute natural favorites such as cheese, meat, and fish, consumers find assessing nutritional value difficult. We need labels that everyone can understand. In cases where it would be cumbersome to attach a label containing nutritional information to a food product (for example, a cinnamon bun baked in the store), the nutritional breakdown could be provided by the cashier at point-of-purchase.

So who is responsible for our food labels? The state departments/ministries of health, agriculture, food, and rural affairs are chiefly responsible for developing nutritional labeling systems. If you're not happy with food labels, contacting these departments/ministries, as well as the product manufacturers, can help to bring about changes in the way nutritional information is presented.

Making Sense of Labels

Nutritional information on food labels must make sense. It's not enough that labels are written in plain English; they need to address the dietary concerns of consumers.

For example, since 1993 in the United States, food labels have been adhering to strict guidelines set out by the Food and Drug Administration (FDA) and the U.S. Department of Agriculture's (USDA) Food Safety and Inspection Service (FSIS). All labels list "Nutrition Facts" on the side or back of the package. The "Percent Daily Values" column tells you how high or low that food is in various nutrients, such as fat, saturated fat, and cholesterol.

A number of 5 or less is "low"—good news if the product shows <5 for fat, saturated fat, and cholesterol—bad news if the product is <5 for fiber. Serving sizes are also confusing. Foods that are similar are given the same type of serving size defined by the FDA. That means that five cereals that all weigh X grams per cup will share the same serving sizes.

Calories (how much energy) and calories from fat (how much fat) are also listed per serving of food. Total carbohydrate, dietary fiber, sugars, other carbohydrates (i.e., starches), total fat, saturated fat, cholesterol, sodium, potassium, vitamins, and minerals are given in Percent Daily Values, based on the 2,000-calorie diet recommended by the U.S. government. (In Canada, Recommended Nutrient Intake (RNI) is used for vitamins and minerals, while ingredients on labels are listed according to weight, with the "most" listed first.)

But that's not where the confusion ends—or even begins! You have to wade through the various claims and understand what they mean. For example, anything that is "X"-free (as in sugar-free, saturated fat-free, cholesterol-free, sodium-free, calorie-free, and so on) means that the product indeed has "no X" or that "X" is so tiny, it is dietarily insignificant. This is not the same thing as a label that says "95 percent fat-free." In this case, the product contains relatively small amounts of fat, but still has fat. This claim is based on 100 grams of the product. For example, if a snack food contains 2.5 grams of fat per 50 grams, it can be said to be "95 percent fat-free."

A label that screams "low in saturated fat" or "low in calories" is not fat-free or calorie-free. It means that you can eat a large amount of that food without exceeding the Daily Value for that food. In potato-chip country, it means you can eat twelve potato chips instead of six. "Cholesterol-free" or "low cholesterol" means that the product doesn't have any, or much, animal fat (hence, cholesterol). This doesn't mean "low fat." Pure vegetable oil doesn't come from animals but is pure fat. And then there are the comparison claims such as "fewer," "reduced," "less," "more," or "light" (or worse, "lite"). These words appear on foods that have been nutritionally altered from a previous version or a competitor's version. To be light or "lite" a product has to contain either one-third fewer calories or half the fat of the regular product. Or, a low-calorie or low-fat food contains 50 percent less sodium. Something that is "light" in sodium means it has at least 50 percent less sodium than the regular product, such as canned soup.

When a label says sugar-free, it contains less than 0.5 grams of sugar per serving, while a "reduced-sugar" food contains at least 25 percent less sugar per serving than the regular product. If the label also states that the product is not a reduced or low-calorie food, or it is not for weight control, it's got enough sugar in there to make you think twice. But sugar-free in the language of labels simply means sucrose-free. That doesn't mean the product is carbohydrate-free, as in dextrose-free, lactose-free, glucose-free, or fructose-free. "No added sugar," "without added sugar," or "no sugar added" simply means: "We didn't put the sugar in, Nature did." Again, reading the number of carbohydrates on the nutrition information label is the most accurate way to know the amount of sugar in the product.

New labels have entered the marketplace in the last couple of years. As of 2006, for example, trans fats are now listed, along with saturated fats and cholesterol on the nutrition facts labels.

Food Deserts and Poverty

Poverty is an enormous barrier to a healthy diet and lifestyle, and while the problem used to be particularly rampant in the elder community, it is now more of a problem in single mother–led families. A 2007 report from the Center for Urban Economics, based in Dallas, notes in its introduction: "Many of us take for granted that there are grocery stores in our neighborhoods selling a wide variety of nutritious foods at relatively low cost." This paper focused on the problem of "food deserts," in which access to reasonably priced, nutritious food is a much more difficult problem than is commonly recognized, "affecting more than 400,000 residents in Dallas County, Texas." Sadly, this is just one example in one city in the United States. Because they may not have the money to spend on transportation, many low-income families shop for food at small convenience stores where the quality and selection of healthy food products, such as fresh vegetables, are limited. Ironically, convenience store prices are generally higher than those at suburban grocery stores. Transportation barriers also exist for the disabled, which, again, limit to your diet grocery shopping locations. And since poverty and poor literacy skills often go hand in hand, complicated nutrition labels can be a real barrier to accessing healthy foods.

If you live in a food desert, here are some things you can do to help put more nutritious foods into your local grocery store:

- Together with others in your community who share the same problem, look into alternative methods of shopping or eating through community kitchens, food-buying clubs, and networking with farmers, who may be willing to do "field-to-table programs." You could also start a community garden.

- Contact food manufacturers and encourage them to donate all unused fresh produce and other healthy foods to food banks or community kitchens.
- If you're a parent, get your school board to institute a school breakfast and/or lunch program to help children in need eat more nutritiously.
- Contact your city planning department and let them know that your community is in need of good food stores rather than convenience stores.
- In economically strapped communities, it might be worthwhile to contact some of the larger food stores with good selections and encourage them to invest in your community by buying out some of the deadwood retailers (such as pawnshops or money marts) and opening some new stores. This trend is seen in many large urban centers as part of urban renewal programs.

Marketing Board and Producer Associations

State and provincial marketing boards and producer associations that work with our farmers are an important part of the food production and distribution system. Most of these boards and associations are involved in the quality production of fruits, vegetables, and grains. In the last few years, in response to consumer demand for lower-fat products, the meat and dairy industries in particular are making lower-fat products available. There are also a variety of soy manufacturers who are delivering meat and dairy substitutes in the form of tofu burgers, tofu cheeses, or even tofu turkeys.

Understanding the grading of meat is another problem. For example, in Canada, consumers believe that the highest-quality grades (AAA) are the healthiest, when in fact they are often the fattiest. To meet AAA criteria, meat has to contain greater marbling (visible fat). Beef with no visible fat is graded B; but it may in fact be leaner. "High-quality" beef must therefore revert to its previous status as a high-fat-containing food that could prove harmful to health. So when shopping for meat, be sure to check with your local meat marketing board what your meat grading refers to.

Other Barriers to Healthy Eating

Familiarity with cooking various foods is a huge factor in buying habits. Many people are limited in their tofu or vegetarian recipes, for example, so they tend to buy foods they feel more comfortable preparing. There are also good foods that are only bad when they are cooked in oil or fat; potato wedges baked in an oven, for example, have a much lower fat content than French fries prepared in a conventional deep fryer. Another major barrier to healthy eating is food in the workplace. All community institutions (schools and hospitals) and workplaces with a food services or vending machine should be required to provide healthy food alternatives. Nutritional information about available foods should be posted on the premises, close to where the foods are serviced. One way of enforcing this measure is to demand that nutritional requirements and ingredients lists become part of all catering contracts.

The explosion in pediatric obesity points to the need to begin in the school system.

- *Food education in schools.* We have sex education; why not food education? Suggest this to your school board, which can collaborate with the Department/Ministry of Health and the Department/Ministry of Education to make nutrition education a necessary part of comprehensive school health programs. Our children are being bombarded with commercials on TV that sell them sugar and high-fat snack foods.
- *No junk food in schools.* As a result of pressure from parents, schools have responded, and many have changed their food offerings. If your school is still peddling junk food, get some parents together and demand your school be a junk-food-free zone. The prevalence of foods low in nutritional value and/or high in fat in school cafeterias and vending machines helps to keep our children unhealthy. California has brought in strong bans on junk foods. The law, which went into effect in July 2007, establishes limits on fat and sugar content and portion size on all foods sold à la carte, in vending machines or school stores, or as part of a school fund- raiser. New standards are in place for what types of drinks can be available in school vending machines as well. In 2009 there will be a complete ban on the sale of soda and other sweetened beverages on all high school campuses in California finally occurred.

- *Limit commercial television.* Limit your child's access to commercial television programming for children that is basically a vehicle to sell sugary cereals and junk food. Some foods aimed at children contain as much as 22 grams of fat and 1,500 mg of sodium. Selling pies and cakes as breakfast foods to children raises some ethical questions as well in that it can be argued that junk food for breakfast is harmful.

Avoid Ruining the Right Foods

The American Institute for Cancer Research's Diet and Cancer Project, Food Nutrition and the Prevention of Cancer, recommends that by avoiding the following, you'll decrease your risk of cancer:

- Avoid salted foods and table salt whenever possible; season your foods with herbs.
- Avoid eating food that was left out for long periods of time; the food can become contaminated with bacteria.
- Avoid eating perishable foods that were not refrigerated.
- Avoid unlabeled foods when traveling in undeveloped or developing countries, as contaminants, additives, and other residues are not properly regulated in these areas.
- Avoid charred food, or meat and fish cooked over an open flame.
- Avoid cured or smoked meats. The nitrites these foods contain are carcinogenic.

CONTROLLING ALCOHOL AND PREVENTING ALCOHOLISM

It seems as though one contradictory study after another comes out about alcohol consumption and its link to various kinds of cancer. Alcohol abuse and alcoholism are one of the most common social problems of the past two centuries; but alcohol, in moderation, isn't a bad thing, and even has some health benefits.

One of the most infamous public health failures was Prohibition, which, in the United States, banned the manufacture, sale, and distribution of alcohol. This is also known as the Eighteenth Amendment to the U.S. Constitution (or the Volstead Act), which was passed after World War I in response to extreme conservatism. Prohibition dominated North American life throughout the early part of the twentieth century (some of our grand-parents may still remember it).

What we learned about Prohibition is that it didn't work, and led to un-paralleled drinking of inferior and cruder alcohol concoctions called *bootleg*, which people made themselves. In fact, more time and energy was wasted try-ing to control alcohol smuggling or bootlegging, and other crimes associated with smuggling, using up law enforcement resources that should have been available for more serious problems. The enormous failure of Prohibition led to its repeal, or the Twenty-first Amendment of the U.S. Constitution in 1933. In light of the lessons learned from Prohibition, why do we still want to control alcohol? Well, we still need to prevent moderate drinking from spill-ing over into heavy, addictive drinking, or alcoholism, which causes a number of serious health problems, including certain cancers.

Approximately 10 percent of cancer deaths are at least in part attribut-able to alcohol. Alcohol has been identified as a cause of oral, pharyngeal, laryngeal, and esophageal cancers, especially in those who also smoke. In fact, the lifetime risk of being diagnosed with these cancers is thirty-five times higher in people who both smoke and drink. Alcohol is also a cause of prima-ry liver cancer (common in the aboriginal population), and a possible cause of breast and colorectal cancers. The cancers caused by alcohol are largely pre-ventable, as are the other adverse health, social, and economic consequences of heavy drinking.

One of the problems with lowering alcohol consumption is conflict-ing information about alcohol—especially since there is good evidence to support that alcohol can help to lower cholesterol. For example, it's also been shown that two drinks daily for men and one drink daily for women may lower the risk of heart disease. The alcohol raises your HDL, or "good" cholesterol, thus reducing the deposits of cholesterol in the arterial walls.

So what are the official guidelines for consuming alcohol? The National Institute on Alcohol Abuse and Alcoholism (NIAAA) recommends that for most adults, moderate alcohol use—up to two drinks per day for men and one drink per day for women and older people—is acceptable. One drink equals one 12-ounce bottle of beer or a wine cooler, one 5-ounce glass of wine, or 1.5 ounces of 80-proof distilled spirits. Those with lower than aver-age body weight, or those at significant risk for certain diseases or conditions, should drink less.

When your consumption levels exceed the recommended limits, your risk factor of alcohol-related diseases is higher than it should be, too. Although moderate alcohol consumption might have potential health benefits, for some cancers there may be no safe level of consumption.

Breast Cancer and Alcohol

Since much of the information on alcohol and health is based on studies of men, women are often confused about the link between cancer risk and their alcohol consumption. Using breast cancer risk rules is a good guideline for any estrogen-dependent cancer. As the AICR notes pointedly on its Web site on a page entitled "Should Women Drink Alcohol," basically as a women's intake of alcohol increases, so does her risk of breast cancer: "A woman who consumes no alcohol at all has an 8.8 percent chance of developing breast cancer before she reaches 80. A woman who has one alcoholic drink daily faces a 9.4 percent chance of doing so. Two drinks a day raise the odds to 10.1 percent, and four drinks a day raise her chances to 11.6 percent."

Preventing Alcohol Abuse

Studies have consistently shown that alcohol education aimed at our entire population can reduce the proportion of heavy drinkers and alcohol-related problems. Drinking is, after all, a social activity for many of us. By targeting the entire population with alcohol-consumption education, we can reach anyone vulnerable to alcohol abuse, a problem that is not income specific. Alcohol abuse spans everything from drinking and driving and binge drinking (common on university campuses, for example) to full-blown alcoholism. College and university campuses across North America have recently put strong alcohol policies in place to deal with the problems of student/ underage drinking. To find out more about a campus's individual policies, go to www.collegedrinkingprevention.gov (sponsored by the NIAAA), which offers statistics, summaries, links to colleges, and special links catering to both students and their parents.

Liquor Control Boards

It's long been known that corner liquor stores in large U.S. cities help to breed alcohol abuse. This is one reason why some states, such as Philadelphia, as well as most provinces in Canada, have set up the controlled distribution and sale of alcohol. Ontario is an example of a monopoly system of alcohol distribution, which has been a proven deterrent to alcohol-related problems. In such regions, for example, the state or province controls the sale of a large share of alcoholic beverages in state- or provincially-run outlets, and only licenses establishments that conform with state or provincial regulations.

Controlling access to alcohol, studies show, really helps to reduce consumption. Legislation governing the advertising and promotion of alcoholic beverages, legal drinking age, hours of operation, and retail sales, as well as the number of stores allowed per capita, are good initiatives.

Training the Alcohol Servers

Properly training and educating the servers of alcohol, that is, the staff of licensed bars and restaurants, leads to fewer alcohol-related problems. This training is known as Training for Intervention Procedures (TIPS) in the United States, and Server Intervention Programs (SIPs) in Canada, and involves education about the dangers of excessive drinking, including automobile accidents and violence. TIPS/SIPs help to promote and reinforce moderate drinking as the social norm, and heavy drinking as a social harm.

One of the best ways consumers can support TIPS/SIPs is to ask their favorite establishments if their staff is TIP or SIP-trained. If not, suggest this training to the owner of the establishment. It could reduce the amount of drunk drivers in your area, for example, not to mention lower the health risks associated with alcohol abuse. TIPS/SIPs should become requirements before a liquor license is either obtained or extended.

CHAPTER 4

ACTIVE LIVING

The American and Canadian Cancer Societies state that people who are active have lower rates of cancer. Active people also tend to consume more of the scarce micronutrients our bodies crave. Both of these factors have recently been associated with a reduced risk of cancer. There is evidence that even moderate amounts of physical activity will help to reduce the incidence of breast and other cancers. In the 2007 report from the AICR and the WCRF, *Food, Nutrition, Physical Activity, and the Prevention of Cancer*, are specific recommendations regarding activity and cancer prevention. As noted in this report, physical activity (occupational, household, transport, and recreational) modifies the risk of the following cancers.

- *Colon cancer.* There is convincing evidence that physical activity decreases risk. The evidence is stronger for colon than for rectal cancer.
- *Breast (postmenopausal) and endometrial cancers.* There is probable evidence.
- *Lung, pancreas, and breast (premenopausal) cancers.* There is limited-suggestive evidence.

As of this writing, physical activity is associated with a reduced risk of advanced or aggressive cancer of the prostate, but there is not enough evidence to state a direct association.

Generally, about 25 percent of cancer cases globally are due to excess weight and a sedentary lifestyle. And as far as goes connecting a sedentary lifestyle with specific cancers, the report notes that our occupations have generally become more sedentary; we drive more cars or ride public transport more than we walk places. For children as well as adults, active recreation has been largely replaced by watching television or other sedentary activities.

This has reduced our activity to dangerous levels. Relatively low levels of physical activity, which is typical in high-income countries and in urban-industrial settings, may be directly linked to cancers of the colon, breast (postmenopause), and endometrium. That said, it is difficult to separate out which cancers are linked to obesity, and which to exercise, since they are so intricately linked.

Public health agencies in the United States and Canada have advocated for more active living in communities. Some of examples include bike racks at shops, schools, and workplaces; parks with maintained and accessible trails; workplaces that provide active spaces (e.g., a fitness facility with showers and lockers, picnic tables, a basketball hoop, and walking paths); preservation of green spaces; and the encouragement of active transportation to, from, and at work. These are precisely the kinds of practices put into play in cities across North America. Communities are taking more initiative and have progressively displayed interest in creating healthier towns and cities, more green spaces, and placing more focus on the outdoors and exercise.

In Boulder, Colorado, bicycle commuting is a popular method of getting around, and as the city's official Web site (www.bouldercolorado.gov) states, "GO Boulder strives to develop a sustainable and balanced transportation system that supports the quality of life valued by Boulder's residents, employees, and visitors." On the site are links to biking and walking maps in the city, as well as information on car- and van pooling. A local bicycle commuters nonprofit community group, Boulder Bicycle Commuters, active on both the city and state level, "advocate for safe and convenient bicycle facilities and fair laws for bicyclists." They also work on both on-street and off-street bike facilities, among other things.

The Colorado Department of Public Health and Environment also has developed COPAN: the Colorado Physical Activity and Nutrition Program, which partners in the Denver area with the Kaiser Permanente Thriving Communities Initiative. They worked together to implement the Colorado Physical Activity and Nutrition State Plan, 2010, which, according to the Web site, promoted "healthy eating and physical activity in order to successfully prevent and reduce overweight, obesity, and related chronic diseases." This is an impressive partnership that is being mirrored across the country in other cities and states.

Portland, Oregon, is another U.S. city putting a lot of time, effort, and money into creating healthier and more active alternatives when it comes to transportation. The city's Office of Transportation promotes the program SmartTrips Southeast, which is designed specifically to encourage bicycling, walking, car sharing/pooling, and transit ridership. The city saw a 9.4 percent reduction in drive-alone trips in the area in its first year of implementation. The program also offers materials for sale, including citywide bicycle maps and walking maps.

TEACHING CHILDREN ABOUT ACTIVE LIVING

You don't need to "teach" children to be active; they are born knowing how. We, in fact, teach them to become inactive through allowing them to engage in too many sedentary activities, such as watching television, sitting in front of the computer, or playing endless video games. We teach them inactivity by making them sit at a desk all day (which may not even be the best way to promote learning). We expose them to commercials that sell them sugar in the form of junk food and soft drinks. Studies also show that physical activity is a clear deterrent from smoking and other substance abuse in the teenage population, and may also improve mental health, cutting down on mood disorders and teen suicides.

Preventing Childhood Obesity

Obesity in childhood and adolescence is at an all-time high in North America. Results from the 2009–2010 National Health and Nutrition Examination Survey (NHANES) estimate that 17 percent of children and adolescents age 2 to 19 are obese. North Americans have the highest obesity rates in the world. More than half of North American adults and about 25 percent of North American children are now obese. These figures reflect a doubling of adult obesity rates since the 1960s, and a doubling of the childhood obesity rate since the late 1970s—a staggering increase when you think about it in raw numbers.

As the CDC states on its Web site, the rise in obesity rates is clearly a complex combination of lifestyle, environmental, and genetic factors: "Obesity and overweight are a result of an imbalance between food consumed and physical activity. . . . Many underlying factors have been linked to the increase in obesity, such as increasing portion sizes; eating out more often; increased consumption of sugar-sweetened drinks; increasing television, computer, electronic gaming time; changing labor markets; and fear of crime, which prevents outdoor activities."

The CDC has tracked obesity rates by state, considering gender, age, race, and education level. In 1991, only four states had obesity rates of 15 percent or higher; today at least thirty-seven states do. The CDC study compared the spread of obesity throughout the United States to the spread of a communicable disease during an epidemic. In Canada, the rates of obesity are climbing at an equal speed, particularly in the aboriginal communities and nonwhite populations. Obesity is now second only to smoking as a leading cause of death. In the United States alone, obesity-related healthcare costs are close to $240 billion.

The American National Health and Nutrition Examination Survey III (NHANES III) revealed that 21 percent of people age 12 to 19 were obese (i.e., their body weight exceeds the ideal weight for someone of their height by more than 20 percent), while as many as 40 percent of people in that age group were physically unfit. It wasn't until 1995 that the Dietary Guidelines for Americans even recommended physical activity. The 2005 guidelines recommend that children and adolescents engage in at least sixty minutes of physical activity on most, preferably all, days of the week. It's important to help your children establish an active lifestyle early—one that will lower their risk for chronic illnesses and cancers.

The Role of Television in Creating Sedentary Children

The average child in the United States watches between two and three hours of television a day, consuming high-fat snacks while they're watching the advertising of more high-fat snacks. If you count computer time and other electronic devices as well as video games, children spend more than thirty-eight hours a week in front of some type of screen; that almost equals the hours spent on the average full-time job. Children watch more than 30,000 commercials per year, and roughly 25 percent of North American children between the ages of 2 and 5 actually have a TV in their room. Since the 1980s, we have seen a virtual explosion in advertising to children. Food is advertised more than any other product. The Institute of Medicine (IOM) in the United States reported in 2006 that one-third of children in the United States were obese or were at risk of becoming obese, while U.S. companies were spending $15 billion a year marketing and advertising to children under age 12. The situation got so bad, that the IOM formed a standing committee on childhood and obesity prevention in 2008, which can be accessed here: http://www.iom.edu/Activities/Children/ChildObesPrevention.aspx Fast food chains that offer playgrounds and toys with meals encourage children to crave the product.

There is a direct connection between obesity and television commercials. The more commercials children watch, the fatter they get. Several studies have documented that children who watch television are fatter. Two studies from 2007 confirmed this fact. One, from the *International Journal of Behavioral Nutrition and Physical Activity*, looks at the connection between television viewing (and computer use) and obesity in U.S. preschool children. The results showed that watching two or more hours of TV/videos per day was associated with either being overweight or being at risk. The study concludes that guidelines should be introduced for preschool children's media use. Another 2007 study from the journal *Obesity* takes the obesity/television viewing connection to another level, by discussing the connection between having a television in a bedroom and adiposity in adolescence. The results showed strong reasoning for keeping a television out of a child's bedroom for obesity prevention purposes. Although this clearly connects to diet, I discuss the role of television here because it is a problem that begins with inactivity, which then creates the diet problems. Studies show that replacing television with sports or other active play significantly reduces sedentary habits and exposure to harmful advertising, which then impacts diet and adult habits.

Nearly 70 percent of all foods advertised are fast foods. Only about 2 percent of food advertising is for real food, such as fruits, vegetables, grains, or beans. Regardless of whether fast or real food is advertised, 95 percent of all food advertised to children in North America are foods high in sugar, salt, and fat. Food companies spend more than $11 billion annually in North America on advertising in all media. This has been going on for years, to the point where an entire generation has now come of age under a barrage of fast food porn advertisements. For example, the figures for 1999 reflect that most of the advertising targeting children came from fast-food companies: over $627.2 million was spent by McDonald's in the United States alone, and $403.6 million was spent by Burger King.

Children's nagging for food products has actually been measured and analyzed by marketing experts. For example, parents respond to pleading nags ("please, please please!"), persistent nags (repeating the request over and over), forceful nags (with threats attached, such as "I won't do my homework unless..."), demonstrative nags (tantrums—common in candy aisles at check-out counters), pity nags (the child claims he or she will be harmed or shunned in some way if the product isn't bought), and sugarcoated nags (promises/declaration of love in return for the item). Food advertisers count on the children's market to increase their bottom lines; but our children's waistlines are what really expands. For example, most U.S. children now get about 25 percent of their total vegetable servings in the form of potato chips or French fries.

The problem of television and obesity is so endemic that several universities in the last decade began to create pediatric programs to "teach" children about watching less TV, getting more activity, and adopting a healthier diet. The State University of New York and Syracuse's Children's Center for Nutrition and Exercise are two early examples of universities with departments devoted to these issues for children. Childhood obesity is considered to be at epidemic proportions. Genetic factors play only a small role in this problem. Although 40 percent of children may have a tendency to become overweight, sedentary living and high-fat snacking are the switches that "trip" the obesity gene.

But limiting television time does not stop the sedentariness or the advertising. On top of their TV time, children also spend hours at their computers on the Internet, as well as several hours on a host of screen-related devices. The results of more active screen games, using Wii are not known, but Wii does not replace physical exercise.

Online Targeting of Children

Marketing fast-food online, using a range of traditional web marketing and social networking has only aggravated matters. Used by fast-food companies, online marketing is a powerful tool to obtain personal information about children. As early as the late 1990s. A character on McDonald's web site, for example, encouraged kids to send Ronald McDonald an e-mail revealing their favorite menu item at McDonald's. An entire generation has now come of age with fast food sold to them subliminally or more directly, online.

Many consumer and parent groups began to seek to ban junk food advertising to children under age 7, who frequently confuse the advertisements for programming and are therefore more gullible targets. Parental pressure has worked. In 2012 the Walt Disney Company finally announced that it will begin to ban junk food advertising on several of its channels, as well for other venues.

Other Way We Sold Junk Food to Children

But even if children were never exposed to television or web-based ads, they would be targets for fast-food advertising through promotional links between food and toy companies, and the fast-food industry and Hollywood. Food companies subliminally influence children through the guise of education.

One early trend was to produce counting books for young children to promote arithmetic skills. These books required a parent to purchase brand-name candies, cookies, or sugar-sweetened cereals. The books instructed the children to count using their food item as "tokens" that were placed onto a space on the page; teachers and parents found them helpful. So did the food companies. The children became dependent on the brand to learn to count. These books also included value coupons to purchase more products, and, of course, the brand was pictured on every page. Over 1.2 million copies of the Cheerios counting book sold between 1998 and 2000, no doubt selling more Cheerios, too. Froot Loops and Oreo Cookies were other bestsellers. The Oreo Cookies counting books instructed children to count to ten while the children ate their way down from ten to zero. Advertising is also done by branding dozens of nonrelated food items, such as apparel, which influence children as well. The marketing of fast food is even prevalent in hospitals across North America, including, believe it or not, children's hospitals. A 2006 press release from the American Medical Student Association (AMSA) sounded the alarm that many of the nation's top hospitals are serving patients and visitors fast food. The association cites four in ten university-affiliated hospitals serving brand-name fast food from vendors such as Krispy Kreme, Burger King, and McDonald's. A *Washington Post* story in 2004 noted that "of its 13,000 U.S. locations, about 30 McDonald's outlets are in hospitals, including children's hospitals in Los Angeles and Philadelphia." The AMSA, which is the nation's largest independent medical student organization, urges the expulsion of these types of vendors from hospitals. It is hard to escape fast food in our society, but one would expect that in an institution such as a hospital more of an emphasis would be placed on offering nutritionally sound options.

We know from studies done in the in the late 1980s that children spend huge amounts of their own money on food items. At that time, children averaged about $4.42 per week (which amounted to roughly $6 billion per year). Children also influenced family spending, which accounted to another $132 billion.

65

In 1997, children aged 7 to 12 spent $2.3 billion of their own money on snacks and beverages; teens that year spent $58 billion. By 2009 it was tracked that, children aged 3 to 5 account for roughly $1.5 billion of food sales when spending their own money (allowance usually); they now influence an additional $15 billion. Children aged 4 to 12 spend $27 billion on food, and influence an additional $188 billion. In 2001, it was estimated that teens alone accounted for $136 billion in food sales. The 1999 figure for children's spending on food (which included influencing purchases) totaled $485 billion annually. Children control substantially markets for certain foods: salty snacks (25 percent), soft drinks (30 percent), frozen pizza (40 percent), cold cereals (50 percent), and canned pasta (60 percent).

Steps are being taken in the industry to limit food advertising to children. In 2007 McDonald's, Pepsico, and Campbell Soup agreed to stop advertising to children under age for 12 products that do not meet certain nutritional standards. Coca-Cola withdrew all such commercials but began marketing sugary caffeine drinks, such as Red Bull to the teen demographic.

North American children are considered the worst examples of childhood obesity. Children are now developing obesity-related diseases that were once diagnosed only in adults. Obese children are diagnosed today with type 2 diabetes and high cholesterol; obesity-related cancer could presumably follow if we don't get this problem under control. Between the late 1970s and the early 1990s, the prevalence of childhood obesity had doubled (from 8 to 14 percent in children age 6 to 11, and 6 to 12 percent in teens). Fearing the same fate for their own children, many European countries have taken action. In 1992, Sweden banned all television advertising directed at children under age 12. Advertisements have been similarly banned from children's television programming in Norway, Belgium, Ireland, and Holland. Most countries look at North American children as the "what not to become" example. In 1995 the American Academy of Pediatrics stated that advertising to children under age 8 was exploitative. Although companies doing the advertising assert that banning their advertisements would interfere with their freedoms, child health experts compare the peddling of junk food and fat to our children to peddling tobacco and alcohol to them. Preventing obesity in children means limiting their access to these advertisements.

HOW LOCAL GOVERNMENTS CAN HELP

Urge your local levels of government to promote active living, using Boulder and Portland as living examples. Reports from the Institute of Medicine and of the National Academies are doing a lot to promote the importance of issues of childhood obesity, and the health of youth in general.

A 2005 report, entitled, "Food Marketing to Children and Youth: Threat or Opportunity?" found that "current food and beverage marketing practices put children's long-term health at risk." The IOM makes recommendations to the following groups: the food, beverage, and restaurant industries; food retailers and trade associations; the entertainment industry and the media; parents and caregivers; schools; and the government to promote safe, effective, and healthier advertising strategies to children and youth. The IOM's other reports of interest include can be found at their Web site (www. iom.edu).

SCHOOL-BASED ACTIVITY PROGRAMS

Several U.S. states are taking the issue of childhood obesity and physical activity more seriously. The situation got so bad in Texas, the Texas Association for Health, Physical Education, Recreation and Dance, for example, recommended by the mid-2000s, quality daily physical education instruction be required for kindergarten through grade 12. Texas also passed a bill: Senate Bill 530. The law required physical fitness assessment for all students in grades 3 to 12 starting in the 2007–2008 school year. The Texas Education Agency chose FITNESSGRAM as the assessment tool that will be used by all districts throughout the state. FITNESSGRAM, which was developed by the Cooper Institute, measures three components of health-related physical fitness that have been identified as being important to overall health and function:

- Aerobic capacity
- Body composition
- Muscular strength, endurance, and flexibility

Those who grow up active tend to stay that way. Physical activity is a component of lifestyle, and lifestyle habits need to be established and reinforced throughout the school-age years if they are to be maintained later in life.

Preventing Adult Cancers in Our Children

When it comes to breast cancer, for example, evidence suggests that adverse factors early in life increase the risk, whereas the benefit of exercise in early life continues to work by reducing subsequent breast cancer risk. Make some of the following suggestions to your child's school:

- *Mandatory physical education throughout secondary school.*
  In most school boards, just one credit in physical education is required at the secondary school level. This sends the message that physical education is not a priority and is not valued in society. Making physical education a requirement at the secondary school level, in addition to nutrition or smoking education courses, may do wonders. You don't have to substitute gym credit for other credits; it should be made as mandatory as school attendance.
- *Upgrade change rooms.* The change room is often the reason so many teens drop gym class. Private change stalls and showers can make a real difference for self-conscious teens, gay or lesbian teens, or teens concerned with under/overdeveloped bodies for their age and gender.
- *Deemphasize competitive sports, and encourage "solitary" activities to be given just as much value.* These activities can be walking, hiking, or bicycling.

CHAPTER 5

SUN SAFETY

By simply becoming educated about sun safety, we can prevent most skin cancers. Skin cancer is a common type of *neoplasm*, or abnormal growth of tissue. There are two types of skin cancer: nonmelanoma and melanoma. The American Cancer Societ estimates approximately 65,000 new cases of melanoma annualy, and roughly 8,500 estimated deaths. If recognized and treated, nonmelanoma skin cancers are rarely fatal, although they can be disfiguring. And because they are often treated in the doctor's office, they are rarely registered (or tracked). Yet nonmelanoma skin cancers are almost certainly the most common types of cancers for North Americans of both sexes. Melanoma is often missed and diagnosed too late because early stages of melanoma frequently have no symptoms. The incidence of melanoma is rising in both sexes, largely due to increased ultraviolet (UV) exposure. With the right information about sun safety in childhood, many · melanomas can be prevented, too.

Did You Know?

- Research shows a link between sunburns in children and an increased risk of melanoma and skin cancer later in life.
- Protecting skin from the sun during childhood and adolescence is important in reducing cancer risk later in life.
- Ultraviolet (UV) rays reflect off water, sand, and snow. UV rays also reach below the water's surface.

Source: American Cancer Society, 2004

ANOTHER PREVENTABLE ENVIRONMENTAL CANCER

Skin cancer, like lung cancer, is an easily preventable environmental cancer. Unlike tobacco, however, the sun wasn't always as bad for you as it is today. It has become a serious health hazard due to all of the environmental pollutants that have damaged the ozone layer.

In the past, the ozone layer of the upper atmosphere protected the earth and its inhabitants from ultraviolet solar radiation. The ozone layer is made up of a band of ozone molecules that ultraviolet rays cannot usually penetrate. As synthetic chemicals (such as chlorofluorocarbons) enter the stratosphere, however, solar radiation splits the ozone molecules into oxygen atoms. Some of these atoms then bond with the synthetic chemicals instead of regrouping, as they're supposed to, into ozone molecules once again. The result is a net loss of ozone and an increased penetration of ultraviolet radiation, something that just "wasn't supposed to happen."

Although the international community has responded to the crisis of ozone depletion by agreeing to phase out the production of most ozone-depleting substances, such as CFCs, the ozone layer will continue to thin for at least another seventy years. It is estimated that for every 1 percent decrease in ozone, we'll see a 3 percent rise in nonmelanoma skin cancers.

Skin Cancers

Most forms of skin cancer are caused by repeated exposure to the sun's ultraviolet rays, which are categorized into A and B, known as UVA and UVB rays. The most damage is done during childhood. Evidence links nonmelanoma skin cancer, in particular, to a combination of sun exposure, geographic location, and genetic susceptibility. You're also at greater risk if you happen to be older, male, fair, and freckled, with either blue or light-colored eyes.

The connection between sun exposure and malignant melanoma is not as clear-cut as the connection between sunlight and nonmelanoma skin cancer. Although we do know that repeated sun exposure during childhood is a primary risk factor for malignant melanoma, establishing a direct link has so far proved impossible. As with nonmelanoma skin cancers, your risk of melanoma increases if you have light hair, skin, and eye color, and if you tend to burn easily. Your risk of melanoma increases even more if you have moles, freckles, or red hair. In fact, the incidence of melanomas among fair-skinned populations is rising at a rate 3 to 6 percent higher than that of darker-skinned people. Moreover, higher rates of melanoma have been reported in geographic areas with lower latitudes, such as Australia.

Educating the Grown-Ups

We won't realize the fruits of sun-safety education for about forty years, because most skin cancers are linked to early damaging exposure to sunlight. Before we can properly educate our children about sun safety, however, most of us need a refresher course, because a lot of us are misinformed.

Minimizing Damaging Exposure to the Sun

Guidelines about sun safety from many different organizations, including the American Academy of Dermatology (AAD), all basically suggest the same precautions when it comes to sun exposure. The following prevention and early detection guidelines are from the American Cancer Society (ACS), and should be considered universal sun-safety guidelines regardless of what country you live in.

1. *Limit direct sun exposure during midday.* The sun's rays are the strongest between 10:00 a.m. and 4:00 p.m. If you can, plan your outdoor activities before or after this time. It's easy to remember this time—during these hours, your shadow is shorter than you are! It is best to plan activities out of the sun during this particular span of time. If you are outdoors, protect your skin.

2. *Cover up.* It is advisable that when you are in the sun, keep your clothing on to protect your skin as much as possible. Furthermore, the darker the color the better, as darker colors provide more protection than lighter colors.

3. *Wear a hat.* The ACS recommends a hat with at least a two- to three-inch brim all around. It can protect the areas often most exposed to the sun, such as the neck, ears, eyes, forehead, nose, and scalp. While baseball caps do offer some protection for the front and top of the head, they don't cover both the ears and back of the neck: places where skin cancers often develop.

4. *Use a sunscreen with an SPF (skin protection factor) of 15 or higher.* Sunscreens provide some protection against the sun's ultraviolet rays, and are available as lotions, creams, ointments, and gels. It is important to apply the sunscreen properly, with maximum effectiveness achieved by applying it twenty to thirty minutes before going outside. Using a

sunscreen lip balm is also recommended. Sunscreens should not be applied on babies younger than 6 months, rather they should be dressed in hats and clothing to protect them from the sun. Although the American Academy of Pediatrics does state on its Web site, "If you cannot keep your child covered in the shade, sunscreen can be applied. However, before covering with sunscreen, be sure to apply a small amount to a limited area and watch for any reaction."

5. *Wear sunglasses that block UV rays.* The ACS notes that "long hours in the sun without adequate eye protection increase your chances of developing eye disease." It is not necessary to buy the most expensive sunglasses for good protection. Look for ones that block out 99 to 100 percent of UVA and UVB radiation.

6. *Avoid sunlamps and tanning booths.* Although many people may be under the illusion that sunlamps and tanning booths are harmless, and that they are a "safe" way to tan, that is simply not true. A 2007 study in the International Journal of Dermatology notes that exposure to tanning beds increases the risk of malignant melanoma, especially in women age 45 and younger. The findings reinforced the hazards of tanning bed exposure. Tanning lamps emit UVA radiation, and often UVB, as well. Both can cause not only serious skin damage but can also contribute to possible skin cancer. Health experts advise people to avoid these methods of tanning. To look like you have been in the sun, consider using a sunless self-tanning product, but do use sunscreen with it. For regulations that govern sunlamp products, go to the FDA Web site at www.fda.gov.

7. *Check your skin regularly.* Most skin cancers can be cured, if caught early enough. Get to know your skin! The best time to thoroughly examine your skin is after a shower or bath. Check your skin in a well-lighted room using both a handheld and full-length mirror. The American Academy of Dermatology (www.aad.org) has a detailed page with diagrams of how exactly to conduct the self-exams. Know the location and appearance of birthmarks and moles. Check your skin regularly so you can detect any changes. See your doctor right away if you notice:

- A birthmark or mole that changes shape, color, size, or surface
- A sore that does not heal
- New growths on your skin
- Patches of skin that bleed, ooze, swell, itch, or become red or bumpy

Add to this list medication checks. Check all your medications to see if they can make you oversensitive to sunlight, a common but once considered minor side effect. Did you know, for example, that even the popular herbal suppement St. John's wort makes you more sensitive to sunlight? The American Cancer Society points out that you have to be especially careful in the sun if you:

- Have certain autoimmune diseases, such as systemic lupus erythematosus (SLE, or "lupus")
- Have had an organ transplant
- Take medicines that lower your immunity
- Take oral contraceptives (birth control pills)
- Take tetracycline, sulfa drugs, or certain other antibiotics
- Take naproxen sodium or certain other nonsteroidal anti-inflammatory drugs
- Take phenothiazines (major tranquilizers and antinausea drugs)
- Take tricyclic antidepressants
- Take thiazide diuretics (medicines used for high blood pressure and some heart conditions)
- Take sulfonylureas (a form of oral antidiabetic medication)

Antibiotics, such as those listed above, are classic culprits. Did you know, too, that sunscreens are misused? They are not designed for sun-worshipping, but for minimizing exposure to the sun when you're out doing normal activities. We need more public education to encourage North Americans to adopt sun-safety guidelines. We also need to make sure that parents and caregivers are getting the right sun-safety messages.

How Consumer Power Can Help

Consumers have a lot of power. Here are some ways we can exercise it:

1. Get some other concerned parents together and lobby your school board to do sun-safety education as part of its health education initiatives (right along with antismoking, physical activity, and nutrition education). Seek out resources from organizations such as Sun Safety for Kids (SSK) at www.sunsafetyforkids.org, which is based in California. Dermatologists from this group put together the SSK "Comprehensive Guide to Sun Safety for Schools" that includes information, policy recommendations, and resources. SSK produces educational videos on sun safety, and is currently involved, according to its Web site, in a school policy development program in partnership with the National Cancer Institute.

2. In addition, encourage your child's school to practice sun safety by adopting the following policies:

    *   When the ultraviolet (UV) index is high, schools should plan in door alternatives to outdoor activities.
    *   Grassy areas should replace paved schoolyards. The classic grade school play area is paved with concrete or asphalt, which reflects harmful UV rays. Grass is preferred; trees should be added for shade.

3. Contact your local government and request that more shaded areas be created at beaches and other outdoor public places frequented by children and young adults. There are incentive programs out there for places wanting to invest in sun-protection structures. For example, the American Academy of Dermatology's Web site offers information on its "Shade Structure Program," which grants awards in the amount of $8,000 for the purchase of permanent shade structures designed to provide shade and ultraviolet (UV) ray protection for outdoor areas. This program is open to nonprofit organizations or educational institutions that serve children and teenagers, age 18 and younger.

4. Contact the manufacturers of your favorite brand of sunscreen and suggest they use some of their public relations dollars on sun-safety campaigns that target parents or caregivers of young children.

74

Remind them that by informing the public about how important their product is, they'll sell more product!

5. Contact other sun product manufacturers (sunglasses, sun hats, or visors) who stand to sell more product by selling protection, too.

6. Contact children's clothing companies and request that they design and manufacture sun-protective clothing. One example is Nozone (www.nozone.ca), which advertises itself as a "North American leader in producing sun protective clothing for children and adults. Our products are great for gardening, hiking, biking, kayaking, sailing, jogging, swimming, or just sitting around the pool."

7. Contact the manufacturers of drugs that cause oversensitivity to the sun, and request that they always include the information in their advertising.

Occupational Sunlight

Anyone who works outdoors is being exposed to an environmental hazard: the sun. The list of workers could include agricultural workers, farmers, horticultural workers, maintenance workers, pipeline workers, ranchers, athletes, fishermen, landscapers, military personnel, police, ski instructors, brick masons, gardeners, lifeguards, oil-field workers, postal carriers, sailors, construction workers, greens keepers, loggers, open-pit miners, railroad track workers, and surveyors.

Public-utility workers in Maryland, for example, whose work involves extensive exposure to sunlight, were found to be at greater risk of squamous cell carcinoma, a common type of skin cancer, and actinic keratosis, another common type of skin cancer. A British study also confirmed the cancer risks associated with prolonged occupational exposure to sunlight. In addition to an increased incidence of squamous cell carcinoma and basal cell carcinoma, British outdoor workers experienced all sorts of melanomas of the skin that had been exposed, such as on the head, face, and neck.

To minimize the impact of prolonged sun exposure among outdoor workers, companies employing outdoor workers should join forces with their state departments or provincial ministries of labor to provide sun-safety gear to all outdoor workers (sunscreen and hats, and protective clothing, such as long-sleeved cotton shirts); shaded areas on-site for breaks; sun-safety education about the appropriate use of sunscreen, and how to do spot checks (checking for unusual changes on the skin, which often appear as spots or moles). The American Public Health Association (APHA) undertook an interesting intervention study with U.S. Postal Service letter carriers, and published the data in a 2007 paper in the association's journal. The association examined whether the letter carriers who received sun-safety intervention (called Project SUNWISE) would wear wide-brim hats and sunscreen more often than those who did not receive the intervention. Results of the trial indicated that the two-year sun-safety intervention was successful in increasing and sustaining regular occupational use of both wide-brim hats and sunscreen. The APHA, in its conclusion, recommends that the hats and sunscreen be available at all USPS stations. Furthermore, it states, "Project SUNWISE intervention has the potential to reduce skin cancer risk among the nearly 345,000 U.S. letter carriers and other outdoor workers who are at risk because of extensive UVR exposure."

In Australia, which has the highest rate of skin cancer in the world, the Cancer Council of New South Wales (www.cancercouncil.com.au) offers a detailed online sun-safety guide specifically for people who work outdoors. Included is a checklist for employers to ensure sun protection is actively practiced in their workplace. Online resources for sun safety abound all across the world, and with a little research you can find those most applicable for either personal or professional reasons.

Protective Clothing

There is a real demand for lightweight fabric clothing that can block harmful UV-B rays. Most of us have the wardrobe already, which consists of a wide-brim hat; cotton pants, longer skirts or dresses; and clothing made of a denser weave of fabric, such as cotton.

Many of us, however, find these clothes too hot for very warm summer days. So what's needed are manufacturers of clothing using an ultraprotective, lightweight fabric offering UV protection in designs that will make us want to wear protective clothing. An Internet search will yield many companies that manufacture sun protective clothing. Contact some local designers, retailers, or schools of fashion design and suggest that sun-safety lines be designed and competitively priced so that consumers can afford these clothes. Departments or Ministries of Health can get involved by instituting labeling that designates certain clothing "sun-safe," so consumers know what they're buying.

SUNSCREENS AND SMOKE SCREENS

Most of us don't understand how to use sunscreen properly, or even what the purpose of a sunscreen is. Sunscreens are classified according to how well they prevent sunburn. The higher the number, the greater the protection. They may also prevent sun-induced pigmentation changes, such as tanning, freckling, and sun spots; photodamage at the DNA level; or wrinkling and skin cancer. As of July 2006, one of the newest sunscreens, which had been for sale in Europe and Canada since 1993, came onto the market in the United States as an over-the-counter (OTC) product. Known as Anthelios SX, it is considered a better product for blocking out the harmful UVA rays, and is a combination of three active ingredients, including the new molecular entity (NME) ecamusule. Sunscreens have been shown to reduce rates of actinic keratoses, a type of skin cancer in humans. In theory, this could mean a reduction in the rates of squamous cell carcinoma as well. Some have estimated that if sunscreen is used regularly in the first eighteen years of life, the lifetime risk of nonmelanoma skin cancer would be reduced by an impressive 78 percent. The most important thing to consider with sunscreen is its proper application. As the American Academy of Dermatology notes on its Web site: "Sunscreen should be applied one half hour before going outdoors. Even water-resistant sunscreens should be reapplied often, about every two hours or after swimming, drying off, or perspiring. Sunscreen should be applied generously and evenly so as not to miss any areas of sun-exposed skin. It should be kept out of the eyes, and UV light-blocking sunglasses should be worn."

The problem with commercial sunscreens is that they encourage a false sense of security. Sun worshippers continue to spend hours on the beach, confident that their sunscreens have made them safe. In reality, there are other, more effective countermeasures against skin damage (such as wearing protective clothing and sitting in the shade), but we haven't seen these measures marketed with the vengeance of sunscreen.

Sunscreen Safety Campaigns

Sunscreen manufacturers ought to include information about what their product does and what it does not do in their advertising. Sunscreens are certainly one measure we can use to reduce skin cancers, but they are not the only measure, and the public needs to be made aware of this fact. A number of big foundations and organizations exist out there to assist the general public in gaining a better grasp of sun-safety practices. The Shade Foundation (www.shadefoundation.org) is just one example of a large-scale campaign that is "dedicated to eradicating melanoma through the education of children and the community in the prevention and detection of skin cancer and the promotion of sun safety." It is an impressive site, offering links to numerous school partnership programs, grant possibilities, and fundraising events. There is also the U.S. Environmental Protectional Agency's (EPA's) Sunwise Program (www.epa.gov), which is "an environmental and health education program that aims to teach the public how to protect themselves from overexposure to the sun through the use of classroom-, school-, and community-based components."

Sunscreen advertising campaigns should also include instructions on sunscreen application and usage; at the moment, this information languishes in tiny print on the packaging. Many people forget to reapply sunscreen after swimming, sweating, or showering. Many people do not know how to efficiently apply sunscreen so that the whole body is protected. There is room for sunscreen "aid" products—products that help you get to hard-to-reach places on the back—that can help to evenly apply it. Local governments can help by making sunscreen readily available and affordable to low-income people at local parks and recreation sites. For example, in Australia, sunscreen is handed out at public beaches and outdoor recreational facilities as part of ongoing public education campaigns aimed at reducing that country's high rate of skin cancer. Since people will still be out in the sun (we're human, and we seek sunlight), widespread use of sunscreen ought to be available to everyone.

SUN AND DAUGHTERS

Caucasian women are particularly vulnerable to sun damage because of deeply entrenched messages from the media and our culture about beauty, body image, and the attractiveness of a suntan. (This is in contrast, however, to conflicting messages about beauty for women of color, who are told that lighter skin is more attractive.) In surveys and interviews, Caucasion women admitted that they felt more attractive and thinner with a tan. The motivations for tanning are not unlike motivations for smoking, rooted in body image and beauty standards (see chapters 2 and 3). However, there are safer techniques for achieving a tan that do not involve direct exposure to sunlight.

Although it would be safer to change the messages women receive about suntans and beauty, in the meantime, we need to encourage our daughters to at least look for safe tanning methods. Check with your dermatologist or family doctor about the safety of self-tanning lotions as an alternative to tanning beds and salons, which cancer experts declare unsafe. It's also one reason why the Affordable Care Act in the U.S. is imposing a new tax on tanning salons, which will help pay for healthcare reform in the U.S. An estimated 30 million Americans use tanning beds each year, while 2.3 million are teenagers. The new tax is designed as a similar deterrent against tanning as cigarette taxes are against smoking. The main ingredient in self-tanning creams, dihydroxyacetone (DHA), is well tolerated in topical applications, with the exception that some people may experience an allergic reaction. The most important thing to remember when using a self-tanning product of any kind is that many of them only offer a very low SPF, sometimes around 3 or 4. Therefore, anyone using such a product must take care to apply sunscreen with at least an SPF of 15 to protect against harmful sun exposure. You may think that your applied tan, in and of itself, will be protective, but it isn't.

VACATIONS IN THE SUN

To get the sun-safety message out to the public, consumers should urge the vacation and travel industries to join forces. Tour companies selling sun vacation travel should be encouraged to spend some of their advertising and promotion budget on sun-safety education. Web sites or travel agencies could offer sun-safety pamphlets for travelers. The World Health Organization, for starters, offers a detailed information sheet on its Web site called "Guidelines for Tour Operators: Minimizing risks associated with ultraviolet radiation exposure." This kind of information could easily be incorporated into brochures for travelers. "Sun Safety in the Caribbean" brochures, for example, could be jointly funded by travel bureaus, airlines, package tour operators, and departments/ministries of tourism. Such brochures could include official guidelines for sun safety, as well as reminders for travelers to check their medications for sun-sensitivity side effects. If you're planning to vacation in the sun, bring along plenty of sunscreen with proper instructions for use, and plan alternative activities for peak sun hours.

Hazards of Sunlight Deprivation

No sun, is no good, either! We need some sunlight; and women, in particular, need some sunlight for bone health, because vitamin D is activated in their bodies by a little sunlight, and women are more at risk than men for osteoporosis. The *American Journal of Clinical Nutrition* addresses this issue in a 2004 paper: "Sensible sun exposure (usually five to ten minutes of exposure of the arms and legs or the hands, arms, and face, two or three times per week) and increased dietary and supplemental vitamin D intakes are reasonable approaches to guarantee vitamin D sufficiency." In another area, a lack of sunlight can result in both sexes (but more commonly in women) in seasonal affective disorder (SAD), a form of depression or low mood that results from being light deprived. Different forms of light therapy can assist people with this disorder.

CHAPTER 6

THE ROLE OF GENES AND INFECTIOUS DISEASES

What is the role of preventing cancer—especially when exposed to carcinogens? Scientists have identified alterations (called *mutations*) in certain genes that increase the risk for various common diseases. This has led some people to believe that having one of these gene mutations means that they will have no control over their risk of developing that disease. This is not true. You can reduce the risk of developing the top killer chronic diseases (heart disease, stroke, and type 2 diabetes) and top killer cancers (lung cancer and colon cancer) by modifying your lifestyle—changing your dietary habits and levels of activity. In other words, your risk for disease is determined not only by your genes, but also by your environment. According to the World Cancer Report, "Environmental factors may modify the cancer risk of individuals affected by inherited cancer syndromes."

If you smoke (see chapter 2), consume a diet that is low in nutrients and high in fat (see chapter 3), drink alcohol to the point of liver damage (see chapter 3), are completely inactive (see chapter 4), or spend hours in the sun without protecting yourself (see chapter 5), your cancer risk will probably increase whether you have a mutation in a cancer gene or not. Cancer genes are like the brakes on a car. As long as the cancer genes are functioning properly, they actually protect you from getting cancer, just like brakes protect you from getting in a car accident. At birth, we are born with two copies of each cancer gene, just like having two sets of brakes on a car. A person who has a mutation in a cancer gene has one copy of the gene that doesn't work. It's like having one set of brakes that don't work: you can still drive, but if anything happens to that second set of brakes, you are at really high risk. Certain triggers, such as food, tobacco, or other toxins (see chapters 7 to 10) can damage these genetic brakes. If you have a lung cancer gene mutation, so what? If you don't smoke, you have a much better chance that your normal copy of the lung cancer gene, that second set of brakes, won't go out.

This chapter takes a closer look at what having mutations in certain genes means. It also explores the issue of genetic testing as a way identifying people at increased risk for cancer, so that they can make lifestyle choices that can help stop cancers before they start.

THE ROLE OF GENES IN CANCER

We are now certain that most cancers occur because of changes in the genetic makeup of cells that cause them to become cancerous. The genes involved in cancer are normal genes that have both tumor-causing and tumor-suppressing functions. In other words, these are normal genes that can be altered by cancer-causing substances called *carcinogens*, such as tobacco.

All cancers involve the malfunction of genes that control cell growth and division. About 5 to 10 percent of all cancers are due to a strong hereditary risk, which means in that an inherited gene mutation confers a high risk of developing one or more specific types of cancer. However, most cancers do not result from gene mutation that a person is born with, but instead result from the gene mutations that occur during the course of a person's life. Mutations sometimes result from internal factors, such as hormones or spontaneous genetic mutations that occur when a cell makes a mistake in copying its genetic information when it divides. Mutations can also occur due to external factors such as tobacco, chemicals, and UV radiation from sunlight.

Most experts believe cancers are triggered by an interaction between genes and lifestyle habits (smoking, drinking, eating, exercise, and sun exposure habits), as well as other environmental exposures (meaning the air and water around us that we cannot control). When it comes to preventing cancer, the challenge is constantly recognizing the factors in our personal lives and our environment that need to be modified, avoided, or eliminated to ensure that genetic damage and resulting cancers do not occur.

What Common Cancers Are Genetic?

Inherited mutations in these genes are associated with some common cancers.

Gene	Location	Associated Tumors
BRCA1	17q	Breast, Ovary, Prostate
BRCA2	13q	Breast, Ovary, Pancreas, Melanoma, Prostrate
p16	9p	Melanoma, Pancreas
MLH1	3p	Colorectal, Uterus, Ovary
MSH2	2p	Colorectal, Uterus, Ovary
MSH6	2p	Colorectal, Uterus, Ovary
PMS2	7p	Colorectal, Uterus, Ovary

Source: WHO/IARC 2003 World Cancer Report, page 73.

Studies have shown that breast and ovarian cancer often show up over many generations in one family. An inherited mutation in the BRCA1 or BRCA2 gene that increases a women's risk of developing breast cancer increases her risk of ovarian cancer as well. As a result, the two risks are often estimated together. Colon cancer is another type of cancer that is often seen in members of the same family. Gene mutations associated with colon cancer also increase the risk for developing other cancers such as:

- Cancer of the uterus
- Cancer of the rectum (lower end of the large bowel that links it to the anus)
- Stomach cancer
- Cancer of the urinary tract
- Ovarian cancer

For just about every type of cancer, there have been reports of families where the cancer risk seems to be inherited. Other cancers that sometimes occur within the same family include:

- Prostate cancer
- Pancreatic cancer
- Wilm's tumor (a tumor of the kidney)
- Retinoblastoma (a tumor of the eye)

- Medullary thyroid cancer (this type of thyroid cancer accounts for roughly 25 percent of all thyroid cancers; thyroid cancer occurs in roughly 2 percent of the general population)
- Blood cancers, such as leukemia and lymphoma

What It Means to "Carry a Cancer Gene"

You may have heard or read about people that "carry a cancer gene." This is not actually what happens when someone inherits a risk for cancer. Most of the genes that are associated with cancer risk are actually tumor suppressors…as long as they are working correctly, they actually protect you against developing cancer. When a person inherits a risk for cancer, they actually inherit a copy of the gene that has a mutation. The mutation keeps the gene from functioning the right way, so that the gene no longer protects them from developing cancer. Cancers are considered to hereditary when there certain features in the family history, including multiple cases of the same kind of cancer in close relatives on the same side of the family, or two or more family members with the same type of cancer diagnosed before age 50, or a single person with multiple types of cancer. Genetic screening can find some of these mutations that are associated with hereditary cancer risk, but what does this information mean?

The Genetics of Colon Cancer

It is known that mutations in colon cancer genes increase the risk for colon cancer, but the presence of a genetic mutation for colon cancer does not guarantee you will get colon cancer, nor does the absence of a genetic mutation mean that you will *not* get colon cancer. Usually, genetic testing of colon cancer genes is recommended only to people who have a personal or family history that is suggestive of hereditary colon cancer. Even then, some people may not choose to undergo genetic testing, either because they do not feel the information would change their medical decisions, or because they feel they could not cope with knowing that they had a mutation in a colon cancer gene.

So what do you need to know about colon cancer risk due to family history of colon cancer? Firs, it is thought that only about 5 to 10 percent of all colon cancer is hereditary, which means the colon cancer is due to a mutation in a colon cancer gene. Another 15 to 20 percent of people with colon cancer have at least one family member with colon cancer. These so-called familial cases are probably not due to a single mutation in a colon cancer gene, but are probably due to a combination of shared genes and environment within a family. The rest of the colon cancer cases, which account for the majority of colon cancer cases, occur in people that have no family history of colon cancer at all.

If you have a family history of colon cancer, do you need to seek genetic counseling and possibly genetic testing? It really depends on the number of family members who have had colon cancer (or other cancers or conditions related to one of the genetic syndromes described below), and the ages at which they were first diagnosed with cancer. In general, the more family members a person has that were diagnosed with colon cancer before the age of 50, the more likely that person is to have a mutation in a colon cancer gene.

Most colon cancer begins with the growth of small polyps, which are small bumps or mushroom-shaped growths, on the lining of the colon. It is not unusual for a people to get one or two colon polyps during their lifetime. Over time, one or more of these polyps may become cancerous. Most colon cancer can be prevented by removing colon polyps before they become cancerous. Polyps usually can be removed when a person gets a colonoscopy. A colonoscopy is a medical test whereby a thin tube with a tiny camera and a light is put into the colon through the rectum, so that the lining of the colon can be seen on a TV monitor.

The two most common hereditary colon cancer syndromes are *familial adenomatous polyposis* (FAP) and *hereditary nonpolyposis colon cancer syndrome* (HNPCC). A person with FAP gets many polyps at a much earlier age than normal. Many kids with FAP will start to get polyps around age 10. By the age of 20, many people with FAP will have hundreds to thousands of polyps. If the polyps are left in place, then a person with FAP has a very high risk of developing colon cancer, usually before the age of 50. Fortunately, the risk of colon cancer can be reduced dramatically, at first by getting annual colon screening to remove the polyps, and then by surgery. People with FAP who have already developed too many polyps to remove when they have a colon exam will have surgery to remove most of their colon.

Although the other common colon cancer syndrome, HNPCC, is not associated with large numbers of colon polyps, the colon cancers that occur in HNPCC usually start from a polyp. Much as with FAP, a person with HNPCC has a very high risk of developing colon cancer before the age of 50. A person with HNPCC also has an increased risk for other cancers, such as cancer of the uterus, stomach, small intestine, or urinary tract. Again, a person with HNPCC can dramatically reduce the risk of colon cancer by getting a colonoscopy every one to two years beginning as early as age 20. Most people with HNPCC will not have surgery to remove the colon because of polyps, but if they develop colon cancer, the surgeon may recommend a more extensive colon surgery to prevent a new colon cancer from occurring. Increased screening for the other cancers associated with HNPCC may also be recommended.

Even if a person does not have one of the colon cancer syndromes described above, they may still have an increased risk of colon cancer because of a family history of colon cancer and/or other risk factors. It is important to share your medical and family history with your doctor so he or she can determine if you are at increased risk of colon cancer. Your doctor may recommend that you get colon cancer screening more often, and may suggest that you begin before age 50. In addition to reducing the risk of colon cancer by getting the screening recommended by your doctor, studies have shown that people who maintain a healthy weight have a lower risk of several types of cancer, including colon cancer. There are also many studies that show that increased physical activity is associated with a reduction in colon cancer risk. There are preliminary data on proposed diet-related risk factors for colon cancer, such as red meat consumption and fat consumption, as well as proposed protective factors, including selenium, vitamin D, calcium, folate, and fiber. However, additional studies will be necessary to evaluate the accuracy of these associations.

The Genetics of Breast Cancer

Similarly to colon cancer, it is estimated that 5 to 10 percent of all breast cancer is hereditary, which means that the cancer occurs due to a mutation in a breast cancer gene. Another 15 to 20 percent of people with breast cancer have at least one family member with breast cancer. These so-called familial cases are probably not due to a single mutation in a breast cancer gene, but due to a combination of shared genes and environment within a family. The rest of the breast cancer cases, which account for the majority of breast cancer cases, occur in people that have no family history of breast cancer at all.

Who is a good candidate for genetic counseling and possible genetic testing for hereditary breast cancer? Again, your chance of having a mutation in a breast cancer gene depends on the number of people in your family who have had breast cancer (or other cancers or conditions associated with hereditary breast cancer), and the ages at which they were first diagnosed. In general, the more family members a person has that were diagnosed with breast cancer before the age of 50, the more likely that person is to have a mutation in a breast cancer gene.

The most common cause of hereditary breast cancer is *hereditary breast-ovarian cancer syndrome*. Hereditary breast-ovarian cancer syndrome is caused by mutations in one of two breast cancer genes called BRCA1 and BRCA2. A woman with a mutation in one of these two genes has up to an 85 percent lifetime risk of developing breast cancer, with most of the breast cancer risk occurring before age 50. A woman with a mutation in BRCA1 has up to a 60 percent chance of developing ovarian cancer; a woman with a mutation in BRCA2 has up to a 27 percent chance of developing ovarian cancer. These risks can be compared to the 12.5 percent lifetime risk of breast cancer and 1 to 2 percent lifetime risk of ovarian cancer observed in the general population.

A woman with a BRCA1 or BRCA2 mutation has many options for early cancer detection and cancer prevention. For early cancer detection, it is rec-ommended that women with these mutations receive annual mammograms and annual screening breast MRIs beginning no later than age 25, and that they receive ovarian cancer screening including annual sonograms of the ova-ries. Women who wish to reduce the risk of breast and ovarian cancer may choose to have their ovaries surgically removed, which reduces the risk of both types of cancer if it is done before menopause. Other choices for breast cancer risk reduction include taking a medication that interferes with estrogen (such as tamoxifen or raloxifene), or undergoing a risk-reducing mastectomy.

Even if a woman does not have hereditary breast-ovarian cancer syndrome, she may still have an increased risk of breast cancer because of a family history of breast cancer and/or other risk factors. If a woman is at increased risk of breast cancer, her doctor may recommend that she start getting annual mam-mograms before the age of 40, and have additional breast imaging studies such as breast sonograms or breast MRIs, and the doctor may discuss the option of taking medication to reduce the risk of breast cancer. The doctor may also discuss modification of other factors that are associated with increased risk of breast cancer, including long-term hormone replacement therapy and obesity.

Family History of Cancer and You

As it turns out, there are hereditary cases of just about any type of cancer, and the information about the genetics behind these cancers could fill an entire book. It is not the purpose of this chapter to fully explain the genetics behind all types of cancer. The take-home message is that it is important for every person to find out if they have a family history of cancer, and to share this information with their doctor. Your doctor should then be able to determine if you are at increased risk for cancer, make well-informed recommendations for cancer screening, cancer prevention, and lifestyle modification, and offer you a referral for genetic counseling if it is appropriate.

IS GENETIC TESTING RIGHT FOR YOU?

First, it is important to make a distinction between genetic counseling and genetic testing. Genetic counseling is when a genetic specialist obtains a patient's medical and family history information, and uses this information to determine if the patient is at increased risk of a genetic condition. Sometimes, but not always, genetic testing may be useful in clarifying the risk of the genetic condition. Part of the genetic counseling session is discussing the option of genetic testing and helping the patient decide if it is right for him or her. Regardless of whether this testing is performed, the genetic counseling session can help the patient understand his or her risk, and make informed medical decisions. In other words, even if a patient does not want to get genetic testing, genetic counseling may still be useful. On a related note, the American Society of Clinical Oncology recommends that genetic counseling always be provided whenever a cancer genetic test is performed.

If a genetic test could be useful in clarifying the risk for cancer, the genetic counselor will explain the genetic test. Most genetic tests involve laboratory analysis of a sample of blood, and results are usually available within two to eight weeks. The counselor should also discuss the potential advantages and disadvantages of genetic testing.

Some potential advantages to genetic testing:

- It may clarify the risk for cancer.
- It may provide information to make informed medical decisions.
- It may provide an explanation for why cancer occurred.
- It may provide the option of predictive genetic testing for family members.

Some potential disadvantages to genetic testing:

- The test may not be informative, and may not clarify risk of cancer.
- A person may not be able to cope with knowing about a mutation.
- A person may be falsely reassured by a normal result (since he or she still has an average risk of developing cancer).

In addition to the potential advantages and disadvantages of genetic testing itself, there is a laundry list of potential barriers that may prevent someone from pursuing genetic testing:

Cost
The fee for a genetic test can be very expensive if it is not covered by insurance, or if a person does not have insurance. As of this writing, the cost of genetic testing for mutations in BRCA1 and BRCA2 is just over $3,000. Fortunately, the majority of private insurers provide coverage of genetic testing if it is medically necessary, and Medicare covers certain types of cancer genetic testing. Unfortunately, many cancer genetic testing labs do not have contracts with state Medicaid agencies, so most Medicaid patients do not have coverage for cancer genetic testing. In addition, the high cost of cancer genetic testing puts it out of reach for most individuals who do not have insurance.

Access
Although access is not usually an issue for people who have private health insurance, even they may not seek genetic counseling because of lack of information or misinformation about the potential benefits of genetic counseling, or simply because they are geographically distant from a genetic specialist. On a broader level, there are economic factors that limit access to genetic testing, since patients who are uninsured or covered by Medicaid have limited access because of the cost of testing.

Concerns Regarding Confidentiality
Despite the existence of federal legislation (HIPAA) that makes it illegal for your healthcare providers to release your medical information to a third party without your prior written consent, some people still fear that this information may be available to insurers. Although it is unlikely, it is formally possible that this information may be inadvertently released to a third party.

Also, there may be some situations where it is determined that the information should be released to at-risk family members because of duty to warn about certain genetic risks, in spite of HIPAA.

Fear of Genetic Discrimination

Probably the most highly publicized issue regarding cancer genetic testing is the potential for genetic discrimination. This fear is largely ungrounded. First, most states have laws that prohibit genetic information from being used by medical insurers to deny coverage, change terms, or increase individual premiums for individuals with group insurance, and comprehensive federal legislation (Genetic Information Nondiscrimination Act), which provides the same protection both for people with group insurance and those with individual coverage, was just passed earlier this year. Second, there is little evidence that medical insurers, currently or historically, have discriminated against policy holders on the basis of cancer genetic information. However, this does not guarantee that laws will not change in the future, or that insurers will not change their stance on genetic information. In addition, there is no legislation to prevent other entities, such as life insurance companies or long-term care insurers, from potentially using genetic information for policy determination.

It is important to research issues such as these to assure appropriate, ethical, and equitable utilization of genetic testing. Research institutes, such as the NIH's National Human Genome Research Institute (NHGRI), have research programs specifically to deal with the ethical, legal, and social implications not only for genetic testing in cancer but also for a myriad of other diseases. The ELSI Ethical, Legal, and Social Implications Research Program was established in 1990 as an integral part of the Human Genome Project (HGP) to foster basic and applied research on the ethical, legal, and social implications of genetic and genomic research for individuals, families, and communities. The ELSI Research Program funds and manages studies, and supports workshops, research consortia, and policy conferences related to these topics. The NHGRI's Web site (www.genome.gov) offers links to numerous papers and research reports specifically on the timely topics of genomic medicine, the notion of needing to balance research with ethics, and what changes the era of genomics will ultimately bring to the world of health care. These and other documents are available at the NHGRI site.

The Bottom Line on the Genetics of Cancer

Your family history may put you at increased risk for cancer. Your doctor can determine whether you should be referred for genetic counseling, and the genetic counselor can help you decide if genetic testing is right for you. Ultimately, the goals are to inform yourself about the effect your family history has on your risk for cancer, and to use this information to make positive changes that maximize early detection and prevention of cancer.

INFECTIOUS DISEASES AND THE LINK TO CANCER

Infectious diseases are caused by exposure to microorganisms such as bacteria, viruses, and parasites. It's now known that about 20 percent of cancers are caused by infectious microorganisms. The following is a list of known infectious diseases linked to specific cancers:

- HTLV-1 has been linked to adult T-cell leukemia/lymphoma.
- Helicobacter pylori (H. pylori) bacteria increase a person's risk of stomach cancer, although most people who develop ulcers as a result of Helicobacter pylori never develop cancer.
- Hepatitis. Chronic hepatitis B and hepatitis C viruses are known to cause liver cancer in some cases.
- HIV (See next section)
- HPV (See further)
- Gonorrhea. Some studies are showing that men with a history of gonorrhea have an almost twofold increased risk of bladder cancer. The association was stronger for invasive and advanced bladder cancer, and among current smokers.

HIV/AIDS and Cancer Risk

The human immunodeficiency virus (HIV) itself plays a role in how cancer grows in people who are HIV-positive. HIV attacks the immune system, which protects the body from infections and disease. A weaker immune system is less able to fight off cancer. People with HIV often have weakened immune systems, which means they will have a greater chance of getting cancer. Some other reasons HIV is associated with cancer include:

- *Greater life expectancy.* People with HIV and acquired immunodeficiency syndrome (AIDS) are living longer. HIV medications are helping people with HIV live longer, healthier lives. But their immune systems do not get fully healthy. As people with HIV live longer, their chances of having other health problems, such as cancer, increase.
- *Greater susceptibility to cancer-causing viruses.* Having HIV and a weakened immune system makes is easier for cancer-causing viruses to stay alive in your body. Once cancer starts in people with weakened immune systems, it grows faster than in healthy people. Some of these viruses include hepatitis B and hepatitis C; and human papillomavirus (see further). Herpes and Epstein-Barr virus (EBV) may also be associated with certain cancers.
- *Smoking-related.* About 60 to 70 percent of people with HIV smoke. Smoking is a risk factor for many different types of cancer. As people with HIV live longer and continue to smoke, they increase their risk of developing smoking-related cancers.

In multiple studies, it's shown that circumcising men can significantly reduce sexually transmitted infections, including HIV and HPV, which can eventually lead to sexually-transmitted related cancers in populations where condom use is low. For example cancer of the penis is almost unheard of in circumcised men. Circumcision is preferable in newborn baby boys, but it can be done at any age, with few complications when done by a trained expert.

HIV-Related Cancers

In the past, people with HIV often got three types of cancer: Kaposi's sarcoma, non-Hodgkin's lymphoma, and cervical cancer (in women). These are called AIDS-related cancers because they occur more often in people whose immune systems have been weakened by HIV/AIDS.

Kaposi's sarcoma (KS) grows into reddish-purple patches on your skin that cannot kill you. It can be deadly if it gets in your throat or lungs. A herpes virus causes Kaposi's sarcoma.

Non-Hodgkin's lymphoma usually starts in the lymph glands, which are part of your immune system and help fight off disease. Lymph glands are mainly in the neck, under the arms, in the groin, and inside the belly. Epstein-Barr virus is a risk factor for this cancer.

As for cervical cancer, almost all women who get cervical cancer also have HPV. Having HIV and HPV makes cervical cancer grow faster. Higher incidences in the following cancers in HIV-positive individuals have been observed: anal cancer; Hodgkins lymphoma; liver cancer; cancers of the lip (smokers only) and mouth (smokers only); pharynx (smokers only); trachea, lung (smokers only), and bronchus.

For more information on HIV-related cancers, visit *The Body: The Complete HIV/AIDS Resource*, which can be accessed at www.thebody.com/Forums/AIDS/Cancer/index.html and www.thebody.com/Forums/AIDS/Cancer/index.html.

It's now been shown that highly active antiretroviral therapy (HAART) may prevent most excess risk of KS and non-Hodgkins lymphoma, but not that of Hodgkins lymphoma and other non-AIDS-defining cancers.

Cervical Cancer and Human Papillomavirus

The most well-publicized link between infection and cancer can be seen with cervical cancer. The sexually transmitted disease known as human papillomavirus (HPV) has been clearly linked to causing cervical cancer. HPV is also linked to other cancers of the genital area, mouth, and throat.

There are about one hundred different types of HPV. Some of these cause the common warts found on hands and feet. Other low-risk HPV types cause warts in the genital area or around the anus in both men and women. These warts appear as painless, flesh-colored bumps on the skin. There may be just a few small bumps, or warts can be quite large growths.

A few types of HPV—especially high-risk types 16 and 18—can cause cancer of the cervix in women. They are also linked to cancer of the penis in men, although this is quite rare. Cervical cancer is detected in more than 12,000 women in the United States, and more than 4,000 women die of it each year. This number was higher before Pap smears became a common screening test for cervical cancer. The cervix is the bottom part of the uterus, which forms a canal between the uterus and the vagina. Pap smears are usually done as part of a routine pelvic examination. A sample of cells from the cervix is taken. In a laboratory, the cells are examined for abnormalities. There are several types of abnormal cervical cells. Depending on the type of abnormality, healthcare providers may recommend treatment, taking a closer look (colposcopy and biopsy) or retesting with another Pap smear in several months. Many abnormalities resolve on their own without treatment. However, some abnormalities may progress into cervical cancer, so careful monitoring is important. In the last few years, testing for high-risk types of HPV has been done for some women who have abnormal Pap smears. This can help clarify whether the abnormal cervical cells are due to a low-risk HPV type, in which case cancer is unlikely, or a high-risk HPV type, in which progression to cancer is more likely. For women who have cancerous or precancerous cells (called *dysplasia*) seen on a Pap smear, this HPV typing is not necessary since it is assumed that they have a high-risk HPV type. There are several types of treatment for cervical dysplasia: cryotherapy, electrosurgical excision, a cone biopsy, or laser treatment.

The HPV Vaccine

There is now an HPV vaccine that is recommended to certain populations to prevent cervical cancer. Cervarix and Gardasil are recombinant vaccines against HPV. Cervarix targets HPV-16 and -18, which are responsible for 70 percent of cervical cancers. Gardasil targets the same HPV types, but also targets HPV-6 and -11, responsible for more than 80 percent of genital warts. The American Cancer Society recommends the following guidelines be used for the HPV vaccine:

- Routine HPV vaccination should be given to girls age 11 to 12.
- Girls age 9 may be vaccinated.
- HPV vaccination is recommended for young women age 13 to 18 to catch up missed vaccines or complete the vaccination series.
- Insufficient data exists for recommending routine vaccination for women age 19 to 26; this should be an informed decision by the woman after being counseled about risks/benefits by her doctor.
- HPV vaccination is not recommended for women over 26 or for males at all.
- Pap screens should be done on both vaccinated and unvaccinated women.

Chronic Inflammation and Cancer

Evidence follows chronic inflammation can also cause cancer. Many infectious diseases cause chronic inflammation. This link has been seen with cancers of the cervix, stomach, colon, liver, and bladder as well as some lymphomas. It is also well accepted that chronic inflammation affects the prognosis of cancer, but no one knows exactly why. For this reason, many cancer trials now involve inhibitors of inflammation such as the non-steroidal anti-inflammatory drugs and the cyclooxygenase (Cox-2) inhibitors in dozens of cancer sites.

Inflammation and Prostate Cancer

The case for inflammation can be seen with prostate cancer. Prostate cancer is linked to chronic inflammation of the prostate gland (prostatitis), which is linked to infectious diseases (sexually transmitted diseases). It's suspected that the potential of the infection is to establish a chronic active inflammation. Chronic prostatitis often has no symptoms, but is a frequent cause of elevated blood PSA levels.

CHAPTER 7

OUR BODIES, OUR HOMES: EXPOSURES WE CAN AVOID

Every day, our bodies are exposed to various chemicals and toxins through personal care products and cleaning products. In many cases, there is such a dearth of scientific proof regarding the danger of many of these chemicals that there are no guidelines or consensus reports to use. Many sections in this chapter are based on the peer-reviewed literature to address what we know so far. You can also look at the suspected "body burden" by visiting the Environmental Working Group Web site at www.ewg.org.

COSMETICS AND CANCER RISK

For the last decade, concern has been growing over the risk of cancer from cosmetics. The working theory is that chemicals applied in body care cosmetics (including moisturizers, creams, sprays, or lotions applied to underarm, chest, or breast areas) may be affecting breast cancer incidence in women. The specific cosmetic type is not as important as the chemical ingredients in the formulations, and where on the body these chemicals are applied. The most common chemicals used in body care are p-hydroxybenzoic acid esters, known as *parabens*, which have been shown to be estrogenic in the body, and have now been detected in human breast tumor tissue, indicating absorption by the body.

What We Know—and Still Don't Know—About Parabens and Cancer Risk

Parabens have been used for fifty years in cosmetics, food, and other consumer products. In cosmetics, they are used in a variety of products designed to be applied to the skin, particularly the underarm and breast, and include moisturizers and body lotions. Parabens have antimicrobial and preservative properties, meaning that they have a long shelf life. Parabens are readily absorbed through the skin and gastrointestinal tract, so we do know they seep into our bodies through the skin.

97

There has been almost no progress made in the scientific world toward establishing whether parabens are a conclusive cancer risk. With respect to all estrogen disrupters, such as parabens, the statement that there is "no evidence" that human health is adversely affected is true, because there is no evidence; the appropriate scientific work has not been done. There is enough concern about parabens, however, to *hypothesize* that it may be a problem. Parabens are common in underarm and body care cosmetics, but it is not the type of cosmetic, rather the ingredients in the cosmetic that matter, as well as *where on the body these chemicals are applied*. We worry about parabens because of their ready absorption through the skin, their hormonal activity, and their reproductive toxicity. We also worry that in underarm products, chemicals can affect the lymphatic drainage of the breast, since this drainage goes through the underarm area.

There is limited evidence in the epidemiological world that links underarm cosmetics and breast cancer in women, but that is because study designs haven't been ideal. Similarly, a causal link between cosmetics containing parabens used on the underarm or adjacent body areas and breast cancer has not been established, either.

What We Know So Far

A 1995 study analyzed 215 cosmetic products and found 77 percent of the products investigated contained parabens. The study found that nearly all (99 percent) of the leave-on products and 77 percent of rinse-off products contained parabens. When the products were analyzed for chemicals that should not be present in the moisturizers, according to the manufacturers, at least one chemical was detected in 17 percent of formulations. This suggests that quality control is poor. In light of the problems with quality control on the variety of products now made in China or elsewhere, this problem is likely magnified. In Europe, there is an EC Cosmetics Directive that mandates clear ingredient labeling. More recent surveys of body care products have continued to show that products do not comply with the EC Cosmetics Directive for labeling, and that incorrect ingredient labeling with respect to paraben content was found in 10 percent of investigated products, and that a total of 45 percent of the investigated skin creams had incorrect labeling and that parabens were used extensively, with one or more parabens found in 87 percent of the investigated products.

A 2002 study tried to examine if antiperspirants or deodorants affected breast cancer incidence. This was a population-based, case-controlled study to investigate the relationship between the use of products applied for underarm perspiration and the risk of breast cancer in women age 20 to 74 years, by retrospective interview of 813 case patients and 793 controls. This study reported *no* increase in the risk of breast cancer following the use of anti-perspirants/deodorants and no effect from shaving. A 2003 study found the opposite. The 2003 study found dramatically earlier ages of onset (measured by age of diagnosis) of breast cancer in women who use underarm antiperspirants/deodorants. This study was based on a survey of 437 women diagnosed with breast cancer and gave a detailed analysis, examining the age of starting the use of products and shaving, as well as the intensity or frequency of hygiene/grooming practices. Both the frequency and earlier age of starting the use of antiperspirants/deodorants with underarm shaving were associated with an earlier age of breast cancer diagnosis (differences in age between frequent users and nonusers was in the range 14.7 to 22 years. So the 2003 results clearly suggest a chemical exposure dose–response effect (although specific toxic agents were not identified) and critical sensitivity at a younger age of exposure.

Parabens have also been detected in human breast tumors. That is why we know there is reason to worry. The strongest supporting evidence for a role for underarm cosmetics in breast cancer comes from published clinical observations dating back decades and showing a disproportionately high incidence of breast cancer in the upper outer quadrant of the breast, which some believe simply means that the right-handed nature of a majority of the population led to a greater application of cosmetic chemicals to the left underarm area.

The Joint World Health Organization and United Nations Food and Agriculture Organization (WHO/FAO) Expert Committee on Food Additives (JECFA) evaluated the paraben toxicology database in 1966 and 1974 on their safety for use in food, which today would include cosmetics. Alarmingly, there has not been an updated review since, and the scientific methods used for the first review are now outdated. Toxicology experts today are calling for a new review, and are pleading for further research, evidenced by review articles that end with subheads such as "A Call for Research."

The Antiperspirant E-mail That Scared Women
A few years ago, an e-mail circulated anonymously to millions of women, warning them about damage to sweat ducts by antiperspirant agents as a major cause for breast cancer. Toxicologists are not dismissing this possibility, but there is still no evidence that would suggest this is a true concern. We simply need more research.

What Complicates Things
It's very difficult to measure people's exposure to estrogen from cosmetics, because of the xenoestrogenic soup we are exposed to in general, from the food chain (chapter 8), hormone-containing medications, soil, air, and so forth. There are so many endocrine disruptors (discussed in part 2) that are part of the cancer risk story that risks from cosmetics may never be adequately assessed for years.

What Does It All Mean?
Right now, we know that estrogen exposure causes breast cancer, and it's logical to worry about exposure to the xenoestrogens (estrogenic chemicals) present in cosmetics. The case for parabens has to do with direct application to the skin, and absorption. But, we don't know how significant these exposures are when it comes to breast cancer risk; we just know that body care cosmetics are a "potentially important source of estrogenic chemicals" that may be associated with the rising incidence of breast cancer in women. Given what we know, toxicologists are united in one question and one solution. The question is, "Are parabens suitable to apply regularly to the skin of the general population?" The solution is, "Let's adopt a precautionary principle approach and tell the public to avoid paraben-containing cosmetics until we know more."

What You Can Do: Adopting a Precautionary Principle Approach
Toxicologists are suggesting a number of reasonable precautionary steps that consumers can adopt today on their own, in the absence of governmental regulations:

1. Read labels, and avoid paraben-containing products. This is harder than you might think, considering that labeling may be inadequate on the part of the manufacturer. The Environmental Working Group's Skin Deep is an online, brand-by-brand guide to nearly 15,000 personal care products, ranking them according to their toxicity. (www.cosmeticsdatabase.com.)

2. Switch to something without chemicals. The Green Guide (www. thegreenguide.com) is filled with tips on alternative personal care and home care products you can use.

3. Young teens and children should be more cautious than adults. There are no indications on the containers of any personal care products about a safe level of usage for children and young teens, but we do know that the younger the person (especially in women), the greater the exposure. Prepubescent girls using underarm products need to be especially cautious.

4. Do not apply personal care products with parabens to broken skin. Women continue to apply them after shaving, a procedure that can cause nicks or abrasions in the skin following hair removal.

5. Stay informed online. The FDA is following this area (www.fda.gov/ Cosmetics/default.htm.)

HAIR DYES

There have been concerns worldwide about a possible increase in the risk of cancer among users of hair dyes. Some aromatic amines contained in hair dyes are carcinogenic in animals and humans. The European Union's Scientific Committee on Cosmetic Products and Non-food Products called for an urgent review of this issue in 2004, and concluded that there may be a higher risk of bladder cancer caused by arylamines in hair dyes. There is no agreement that hair dyes cause cancer. The International Agency for Research on Cancer has stated that there is "inadequate evidence of carcinogenicity" of hair dyes. A 2005 meta-analysis, published in *JAMA*, concluded that there is no effect of personal hair dye use on the risk of breast and bladder cancer, but there may be a small increase of hematopoietic cancers.

The use of some dye ingredients, such as 2,4-diaminotoluene and 2,4

-diaminoanisole, was discontinued in the mid-1970s after they were found to be carcinogenic in rodents. But the majority of the studies on hair dyes and cancer were carried out several years after these chemicals were banned from hair dyes. The 2005 meta-analysis found that fewer than half of the hair dye studies done adjusted for smoking, which could also pollute the existing data on hair dyes and cancer. People who work with hair dyes in an occupational setting may be the most appropriate group to study, but this has not been done. The bottom line is that the jury is still out on the hair dye issue, but there is no data that can reliably tell us this is a cancer risk yet.

DRY-CLEANING YOUR CLOTHES

Perchloroethylene—also known as perc, PCE, tetrachloroethyene, and tetra-cholorethylene—is a solvent used in dry-cleaning. Approximately 28,000 U.S. dry cleaners use perchloroethylene, which is the only air toxin emitted from the dry-cleaning process. EPA's Science Advisory Board has identified perchloroethylene as a possible to probable human carcinogen. Epidemiological studies have shown mixed results, with some studies reporting increased incidence of a variety of tumors and other studies not reporting carcinogenic effects.

There is no evidence that wearing dry-cleaned clothing is a significant risk of cancer. There is only evidence that working in a dry-cleaning facility poses an occupational hazard. At this time, dry-cleaning is considered an occupational hazard (see part 2), rather than a consumer health hazard. However, in the absence of any solid proof that dry-cleaned clothing can be toxic to human health, many people will want to adopt a precautionary approach, and avoid dry-cleaning. The Green Guide can point you to other apparel-cleaning options, or fabrics and materials that do not require dry-cleaning.

HORMONE-CONTAINING MEDICATIONS

It's well established that estrogen-containing medications can increase the risk of breast cancers, and other cancers where estrogen receptors play a role. Estrogen-containing medications comprise a myriad of products ranging from birth control to hormone replacement after menopause. Women are currently cautioned against using hormone therapy after menopause for long term, and women who have had breast cancer are cautioned against using hormone therapy.

The guidelines surrounding estrogen-containing medications are highly individualized, and are also based on other risk factors for various cancers. You need to assess your need for these medications with your doctor, and investigate options. For birth control, there are many birth control methods that do not involve estrogen, for example. *No hormone therapy is without risk*, even if the hormone source is derived from plants. Some women suffer greatly from estrogen loss and may want to weigh the benefits against the established risks.

Compounded or "Bioidentical Hormones": What You Need to Know

Many women are turning to compounded, or so-called bioidentical, hormones because they are reading false information on the Internet or in other popular books that bioidentical hormones are "safe" and may even prevent breast cancer. This information is false, and all of the scientific evidence to date points to the contrary that all hormones—regardless of their source (compounded or otherwise)—are a source of potent hormones that can increase a woman's risk of breast cancer or other estrogen-receptor cancers.

The entire compounded hormone industry is also unregulated as of this writing, while the term bioidentical hormones is considered a marketing term, and not a medical term by both the FDA and the Endocrine Society. Proprietors of so-called bioidentical hormones are misleading you when they tell you that such hormones are not a cancer risk.

Testosterone for Men

The risks of testicular cancers or other cancers that respond to male hormone receptors (e.g. prostate cancer) exist when men take testosterone therapies. Abuse of steroids in men is of particular concern, which involves usually young men taking anabolic steroids to improve athletic performance. However, legitimate testosterone therapies can be prescribed for a variety of endocrine disorders in men, where testosterone is deficient, as well as in men who are aging, who may need testosterone therapy to improve libido, and other health factors affected by lower testosterone levels.

Other Drugs

There are several drugs that may block estrogen receptors in some tissues to reduce recurrence of some cancers, but have hormonelike effects in others. Tamoxifen is an example of such a drug. There are also several drugs used in cancer treatment or in the treatment of other diseases, including HIV, which may cause cancers when used in large amounts. In all these cases, you must weigh the benefits of one therapy over the relative risks of the therapy in the short or long term. This book cannot tell you which drugs are a cancer risk, since the risks are highly variable, dose-dependent, and dependent on your other risk factors. A frank discussion with healthcare providers will help you make informed decisions.

Surgical Implants and Breast Implants

There are over sixty case studies showing the development of cancer after foreign bodies or surgical implants are used, but all of these cases are highly individualized, and cannot be generalized to the entire population. The only implant that has been widely and exhaustively studied is the silicon breast implant. To date, studies continue to show that silicon breast implants do not cause breast cancer. Again, informed decisions need to be made regarding the isolated reports of cancers over the benefits of any surgical implants.

HOME-CLEANING PRODUCTS

Another source of avoidable toxic products are home-cleaning products containing formaldehyde, nitrobenzene, methylene chloride, naphthalene, or perclrothylene. Although no cancer has been linked directly to cleaning products, these chemicals are still toxic. There are a variety of "green books" that provide consumers with good alternative cleaning "solutions"—literally and figuratively. Some common homemade cleaners include white vinegar, lemon juice, baking soda, washing soda, and Borax, and some guides recommend olive oil as a furniture polish. Some good sources that provide more information on alternative home cleaners are www.healthychild.org (lots of good tips and recipes for cleaners) and *Home Safe Home*, by Debra Lynn Dadd, at www.dld123.com. (Dadd is a journalist whose body of work revolves around the nontoxic home.)

OTHER EXPOSURES AT HOME

There are a variety of chemicals we expose ourselves to in the home, which include:

- *Cookware.* Nonstick cookware is especially suspect because of questions raise about the toxicity of the surfaces. Use glass, stainless steel, and so forth.
- *Microwave popcorn.* Artificial butter flavors or other flavors now are known to contain chemicals that can be hazardous. Choose natural microwave popcorn without any preservatives or flavors, or just purchase a microwave popcorn maker and use your own kernels.
- *Air fresheners.* Avoid these, and substitute with natural essential oils or homemade potpourri.
- *Carpets and upholstery.* These can contain chemicals and also trigger allergies.
- *Paints and varnishes.* There are now a host of "green" paint products you can use as alternatives.
- *Pesticides.* There are natural forms of herbicides/pesticides, while companion planting techniques from the organic gardening movement can reduce the need to use these.
- *Plastics in the microwave.* When you heat plastics in the microwave, they can leech cancer-causing chemicals into your food. Always microwave using regular ceramic materials or glass.
- *Reduce the use of plastic water bottles.* There has been concern over the use of commercially sold water in plastic bottles because it increases exposure to plastics, as well as contributes to nonbiodegradable waste. Dentists also observe that the rise in commercially sold water has led to an increase in cavities, because people are not drinking as much fluoridated water as they used to.

PRODUCTS FOR BABIES AND CHILDREN

In recent years, alarming consumer reports about toxic toys with lead are a cause for concern. The use of plastic baby bottles is also a concern. Visit www.healtychild.org for alternative products for children that are safe, as well as safe toys. Beware of anything made in China when it comes to products for children, until the regulation of exports and manufactured goods from China is stricter.

Banning Toxic Baby Bottles

In 2008, Canada became the first country to take steps toward a ban on the manufacturing of polycarbonate baby bottles as well as bisphenol A (banned in Canada in 2012) as a toxic substance. Bisphenol A (BPA) is widely used synthetic chemical can mimic the female hormone estrogen. Its use in the manufacturing of baby bottles and in the lining of formula cans places infants at possible risk for developing developmental or neurological problems. When the chemical leeches into the environment, it causes harm to fish and other aquatic organisms.

Polycarbonate is a clear, thick plastic that resembles glass, which accounts for its use in reusable bottles. It can be identified by the recycling symbol of the number 7 in a triangle. Because of growing consumer alarm, many retailers in Canada have already removed polycarbonate bottles from their shelves. (See chart on the following pages for a listing of all products containing bisphenol A.)

Quick-Start Chart—Plastic Products at a Glance

We created this list as a convenient reference to some everyday food storage containers. It is by no means comprehensive! Look for the products you use by brand name, under the appropriate category heading. We encourage you, as a consumer, to identify the unsafe plastics used in your daily life. Other types of plastic food packaging and other plastic items may not be labeled and can only be identified by contacting the manufacturer. We recommend safer alternative materials and practices. By choosing NOT to buy plastics, you send a message to food processors and manufacturers, as well as retailers. Make changes wherever and whenever you can!

A Note on the Food Packaging on Store Shelves

Since so many manufacturers are converting to plastics for their packages, a lot of items formerly available in glass, paper, or metal packages are now available only in plastic! Again, we urge you, as a consumer, to avoid purchasing plastic packaging, especially PVC, PS, and polycarbonate! Choose glass, paper, or metal whenever possible.

Food Packaging and Storage

Caution: Most cling-wrapped meats, cheeses, and other commercially-wrapped foods in delis and grocery stores are wrapped in PVC.

Food Wrap to Avoid
#3 Polyvinyl Films Freeze-tite
#3 Polyvinyl Films Stretch-tite
#3 Reynolds Wrap
#4 Saran with Cling-Plus (formerly Handi-Wrap)
PVDC Saran Classic (formerly Saran Wrap)
#4 Ziploc bags
#4 Glad Cling Wrap
#4 Glad-Lock bags
PVDCGlad Microwave Wrap*
#4 Hefty Baggies
#4 Hefty OneZip Slider Bags
#3 Polyvinyl Films All-Purpose

Plastic Codes to Avoid
#3-PVC
#1-PETE
#6-PS
#2-HDPE
#7-Polycarbonate
#4-LDPE
#5-PP

Cups/ Plates / Utensils Containers to Avoid
#3 Arrow Clearview Pitcher
#6 Arrow Measuring Cups
#3 Arrow Sip-a-Mug (body is PVC, cap is PP)
#3 Arrow Sip-n-Stor cups
#5 Bodum brand plastic cutlery (thick, colored)*
#6 Chip'n Dip bowl (Ullman)
#5 Gladware containers
#7 Intellivent containers with blue lids

Cups/ Plates / Utensils Containers to Avoid
#6 Kingsman Plastic Cutlery (Maryland Plastic)
#3 Marvin the Martian large squeeze bottle (Betras USA)
#5 Playtex Spill-Proof Cups
#5 Playtex Straw Cups
#7 Rubbermaid Clear Classics container bases*
#2 Rubbermaid Pitchers (in colors)
#5 Rubbermaid EZ Topps
#5 Rubbermaid Cereal Keeper
#5 Rubbermaid Servin' Saver
#5 Rubbermaid Ice Cube bins
#5 Rubbermaid Grip 'n Mix Bowls
#5 Rubbermaid Bowl Sets
#5 Rubbermaid Push 'n Pour Decanters
#6 All Styrofoam cups and containers
#6 Sweetheart Plastic Cutlery
#5 Tupperware bowls (all)
#5 Tupperware children's feeding lines
#5 Tupperware Crystal Wave Microwave Container
#2 Tupperware Freeze-N-Save container
#2 Tupperware ice cube tray
#2 Tupperware Ice Tups Set
#5 Tupperware Impressions line
#2 Tupperware Jel-Ring mold
#7 Tupperware Meals-in-Minutes Microsteamer base
#5 Tupperware Modular Mates
#5 Tupperware One Touch Canisters
#5 Tupperware refrigerator and freezer products (except those specified here)
#7 Tupperware Rock N' Serve containers
#5 Ziploc containers

*These items have been discontinued, but may still be found on store shelves.

Water Bottles to Avoid Most 1-, 1.5-, 2-liter (and smaller) beverage bottles are made from #1 or #2
#7 Most 5 Gallon Bottles for water coolers
#7 Appalachian Mountain (gallon size)
#4 Bell Brand Athletic Squeeze Bottles (colors)
#5 Bell Brand Athletic Squeeze Bottles (clear)
#5 Rubbermaid Chuggables bottles
#5 Rubbermaid Sipp 'N Sport bottles

The Green Guide #88/89

IONIZING RADIATION

Radiation has always been a natural part of our environment. Natural radioactive sources in the soil, water, and air contribute to our exposure to ionizing radiation, as well as man-made sources resulting from mining and the use of naturally radioactive materials in power generation, nuclear medicine, consumer products, and military and industrial applications.

Where Does Radiation Exposure Come From?

Here is the breakdown, listed in order of highest source to lowest:

- Radon (43 percent). This is a form of natural background radiation.
- Medical exposure (20 percent): X-rays, and so forth
- Man-made sources (19 percent)
- Earth gamma radiation (15 percent), natural external radiation.
- Cosmic rays (13 percent). This is a form of natural background radiation.
- Food and water (8 percent)

Radon Gas

Radon is a naturally occurring radioactive gas that poses a potential cancer-causing risk. Radon has no odor, color, or taste. It is produced during the decay of uranium, an element found in varying amounts in all rocks and soil all over the world. Radon gas escapes easily from the ground into the air. During its decay process, it can become electrically charged and attach to aerosols, dust, and other particles in the air we breathe. As a result, radon progeny may be deposited on the cells lining the airways where the alpha particles can damage the DNA and potentially cause lung cancer.

When radon gas itself is inhaled, most of it is exhaled before it decays. A small amount of the inhaled radon may transfer from the lungs to the blood and finally to other organs. However, the corresponding doses and associated cancer risk are negligible compared to the lung cancer risk.

Because it dilutes in the air, outdoor radon levels are usually very low. Radon can also be found in drinking water, which can sometimes present a hazard. Radon levels are higher indoors. The highest radon concentrations can be found in places such as mines, caves, and water treatment facilities. Negative health effects from radon have been found in miners. However, the lower concentrations that are found in many homes and buildings, and to which large populations are exposed, also pose health risks. For most people, the greatest exposure to radon comes in the home.

Radon in Homes

The concentration of radon in a home depends on the amount of radon-producing uranium in the underlying rocks and soils, which is how it passes into the home, and the rate of exchange between indoor and outdoor air. Radon gas enters houses through openings such as cracks at concrete floor–wall junctions, gaps in the floor, and small openings in hollow-block walls, and through sumps and drains. Consequently, radon levels are usually higher in basements, cellars, or other structural areas in contact with soil.

The exchange of indoor air with the outside depends on the construction of the house, ventilation habits of the inhabitants, and sealing of windows. The radon concentration in houses directly adjacent to each other can be very different. Radon concentrations within a home can vary with the time of the year, from day to day, and from hour to hour. Because of these fluctuations, finding the average concentration of radon in indoor air requires testing for at least three months and preferably longer. Short-term radon measurements give only limited information.

High radon concentrations have been found in countries where houses are built on soils with a high uranium content and/or high permeability of the ground. In specific geological formations found, for example, in many European countries, radon released from underground waters easily passes through the rock to the ground and into buildings. Many countries around the world may have tens of thousands of houses with indoor radon concentrations above levels considered acceptable.

Health Effects of Radon

The main health hazard from high radon exposure is an increased risk of lung cancer. This has been substantiated in many studies of uranium miners. Based on these studies, the International Agency for Research on Cancer (IARC), a WHO agency specializing in cancer, and the U.S. National Toxicology Program have classified radon as a human carcinogen. Scientists have also been investigating whether levels of radon found in homes and other places are a significant hazard to health. These studies are now complete. The pooled analyses of key studies in Europe, North America, and China have confirmed that radon in homes contributes substantially to the occurrence of lung cancers worldwide. Recent estimates of the proportion of lung cancers attributable to radon range from 6 to 15 percent. The pooling studies all agree on the magnitude of the risk estimates.

When a nonsmoker is exposed to low, moderate, and high concentrations of radon, the risk of lung cancer by age 75 years will be about 4, 5, and 7 in a 1,000, respectively. However, for those who smoke, the risk of lung cancer is about 25 times greater, namely 100, 120, and 160 in a 1,000, respectively. Most of the radon-induced lung cancer cases occur among smokers.

Radon in Drinking Water

In many countries, some homes obtain drinking water from groundwater sources (springs, wells, and boreholes). Underground water often moves through rock containing uranium and radium that produce radon. This is why water from deep-drilled wells normally has much higher concentrations of radon than surface water from rivers, lakes, and streams. More data are needed to better quantify the risk from radon in drinking water.

What You Can Do to Avoid Radon

High levels of radon have been found in all fifty U.S. states and across Canada. Radon testing should be done routinely in all homes. Visit the radon page at the EPA, which is filled with information about testing, how to do it, and so forth. The Web site is www.epa.gov/radon.

Cosmic Radiation

Cosmic radiation is part of our natural environment, and we are constantly exposed to a certain amount of ionizing radiation. Radiation originating from outer space and the sun is called *cosmic radiation* and contributes about 13 percent of the background radiation level on Earth (a greater part is due to radon). Cosmic radiation is a complex mixture of charged and neutral particles, some of them generated when primary particles from space interact with the earth's atmosphere. This complexity also leads to difficulties in measuring radiation doses from cosmic radiation, but physicists have developed sophisticated approaches to deal with this situation. For the human exposure risks, one feature of cosmic radiation is of particular importance: a large percentage of the effective radiation dose from cosmic radiation is due to neutrons of different energy levels. Neutrons are subatomic particles that—when compared to X-rays or Gamma rays—cause more biological damage per dose unit.

Exposure During Flying

As a rule, cosmic radiation levels rise with increasing altitude (up to about 20 km above ground). The actual radiation level is influenced by a number of factors, most important, through the shielding provided by the earth's atmosphere. The overall effect for flight crew and travelers is an increased radiation exposure during flights as compared to staying on the ground. Most flight crew members spend up to 1,000 hours per year on board of flying planes, which leads to annual effective radiation doses in the range of 2 to 5 milliSievert (mSv) for most crew personnel. Occasional travelers obtain a fraction of this value through less-frequent leisure or occupational flights. In comparison, the natural background radiation amounts to 2 to 3 mSv per year at most geographical locations worldwide.

The level of cosmic radiation from flying depends a variety of factors, especially:

1. *Altitude.* The earth's atmospheric layer provides significant shielding from cosmic radiation. At higher altitudes, this shielding effect decreases, leading to higher levels of cosmic radiation. The radiation exposure at conventional aircraft flight altitudes of 30,000 to 40.000 feet (9 to 12 km) is about 100 times higher than on the ground.

2. *Geographic latitude.* The earth's magnetic field deflects many cosmic radiation particles that would otherwise reach ground level. This shielding is most effective at the equator and decreases at higher latitudes, essentially disappearing at the poles. As a result, there is approximately a doubling of cosmic radiation exposure from the equator to the magnetic poles.

Frequent Flyer Exposure

Radiation dose is measured in milliSieverts (mSv). Aircrew flying, say 600 to 800 hours per year, are exposed to 2 to 5 milliSievert (mSv) of radiation each year in addition to the usual radiation of 2 to 3 mSv through man-made (mostly medical) and natural radiation sources on the ground. Aircrew are now recognized in many countries as occupationally exposed to radiation, and radiation protection limits for aircrew are similar to those established for nuclear workers.

Frequent flyers generally do not reach the number of hours flown by aircrew. Thus, unless they fly as much or more than typical aircrew, their radiation exposure and associated possible health risks are likely to be lower than that of aircrew.

Short-haul flights are often flown at lower altitudes than long-haul flights, so that generally, short-haul flights incur less radiation exposure than long-haul flights. An estimate of the radiation dose for a specific flight can be viewed on www.gsf.de/epcard/eng_fluginput.php.

Cancer and Cosmic Radiation

Cancer is the principal health effect that has been associated with low-dose radiation. So far, there is little evidence that occupational exposure to cosmic radiation increases cancer risk. There is only limited evidence that increasing amounts of CR exposure may cause a corresponding increase in certain cancers. Several aircrew studies have shown an increased risk of melanoma and nonmelanoma skin cancer. Solar ultraviolet radiation, such as obtained through suntanning, is an established risk factor for these cancers, but further information is needed to determine if CR exposure also influences the risk. Breast cancer among female aircrew, measured as new illness or related death, was also found to be increased in several studies. Causes other than radiation, such as those from a woman's reproductive history, do not seem to fully explain this increase.

WHO Recommendations Concerning Cosmic Radiation

National governments are advised to:

- Protect flying personnel by law from excessive radiation exposure

Airline management is advised to:

- Assess and track aircrew radiation doses
- Provide aircrew with a record of their personal cumulative radiation dose
- Consider radiation exposure and to reduce occupational radiation exposure where feasible in creating flight rosters
- Inform personnel about the effects of cosmic radiation
- Warn personnel about potential major solar proton events to the extent possible, and advise those who have traveled in an area of increased radiation during an SPE

Aircrew are advised to:

- Keep themselves informed about health effects of cosmic radiation
- Record their personal cumulative radiation doses on a regular basis (if not done by the respective airline or governmental bodies)
- Consider radiation exposure when selecting flight schedules
- Limit flight travels during pregnancy

Frequent flyers are advised to:

- Keep themselves informed about health effects of cosmic radiation
- Limit flight travels during pregnancy

If the flying time of a frequent flyer is similar to that of the aircrew, they are advised to:

- Record their personal cumulative radiation doses on a regular and permanent basis
- Consider radiation exposure when selecting flight schedules

Man-made Sources of Radiation

Man-made sources of ionizing radiation come mostly form medical exposure to X-rays, CT scans, cancer treatment involving external beam radiation, nuclear medicine, and radiation therapy. Thyroid cancer, for example, is treated using radioactive iodine. The public is also exposed to radiation from a range of consumer products, building materials, combustible fuels, televisions, fluorescent lamp starters, smoke detectors, road construction materials, and so forth.

Reducing Your Exposure to Ionizing Radiation from Medical Sources

Therapeutic treatments for cancers, or other diseases, are clearly not an exposure you should try to avoid, since dying from your disease or cancer would be the result without many such therapies. However, there are simple ways you can reduce your exposure to ionizing radiation from diagnostic medical sources:

- Limit the X-rays you have. Many people have unnecessary X-rays. See the X-Ray Record Chart at www.fda.gov to help you assess a lifetime burden of radiation from X-rays.
- Ask that your X-rays are stored on a system that allows other practitioners to access it so you're not having unnecessary duplicate X-rays.
- If your child is being referred for a CT scan or X-ray, check with your doctor and the radiology team that it is adjusted for a child, and not based on an adult dose.
- Discuss with your doctor your routine mammography and adjust screenings to your individual risk factors. Other screening tools such as thermography can be used in combination with thorough breast exams and self-exams.
- If a CT scan is being recommended, see if you can have an MRI instead, which does not involve exposure to ionizing radiation.
- Ask questions of your healthcare providers and weigh the benefits of exposure to ionizing radiation to the risks of cancers.

Other Occupational Exposures to Ionizing Radiation

In addition to airline crews, the following occupations may expose you to greater amounts of ionizing radiation:

- Industrial radiography
- Nuclear medicine practitioners
- Radiology practitioners
- Nuclear power plant workers

PART TWO

WHAT'S POLITICAL

No one in industry or the government woke up one morning and said, "Let's make money and ruin the earth." In other words, you and I bear some responsibility in this mess we've made of our planet. One of the reasons it's so difficult to get rid of many cancer-causing environmental pollutants is that we, as consumers, depend on so many products, which necessitates their production and emissions. I refer to this as our collective "chemical dependency."

The manufacturing of plastic, for example, used in an infinite variety of products, releases carcinogenic chemicals. We need alternatives to the products we've come to rely on, and manufacturers need incentives to create those alternatives. For the sake of our environment, we've had to part with some products we loved. Aerosol sprays, for example, have been removed from the marketplace. We have also largely done away with the production of ozone-destroying chlorofluorocarbons (CFCs), used in refrigeration, air-conditioning systems, and dozens of other products. At first, both consumers and industry members contended that CFCs were irreplaceable, and that stopping their manufacture would deprive us of our standard of living. We screamed, "There are no available substitutes!" "It will cost us thousands of jobs!" But as the ozone depletion problem persisted, public concern helped to eliminate CFCs. By the mid-1990s, the levels of CFCs were significantly reduced in the upper atmosphere, and industry accelerated the phasing out of CFCs in their products. By the year 2015, CFCs will be virtually eliminated, a goal that once seemed impossible. And lo and behold, substitutes for CFCs were developed and replacement products are being made with those substitute processes.

The bottom line is that when given the incentives, manufacturers can be very creative in finding solutions and, in the process, can open new markets and opportunities as well. Indeed, if we can invent ingenious ways to destroy the earth, we can reinvent ways to reverse that destruction. If we can let our voices be heard by government and industry, we can help solve the problems of environmental degradation.

Chapters 8, 9, and 10 discuss the carcinogenic agents that are in our environment—workplace, air, water, soil, food chain—and beyond our personal control.

CHAPTER 8

THE HAZARDS OF WORKING FOR A LIVING

One of the most instructive examples of workplace-related cancers can be seen in the "Bell Cluster." Between April 1995 and September 1996, eight Bell Canada thirty-something employees who worked for the Canadian telephone company, who were hired within similar time frames, and who worked close to one another on the same floor, were diagnosed with cancer: five with breast cancer, two with colon cancer, and one with brain cancer. None of these cancer patients had strong or remarkable family histories of their cancers. The incidence was more than twelve times what would be considered normal in this age group.

This bizarre phenomenon, which seemed to be more than coincidental, became known as the Bell Cluster. These employees (some have since passed away) insisted that their cancers are linked to emissions from their computer equipment, which they said were magnified due to the crowded conditions in which they were working. But since research on the relationship between cancer and electromagnetic fields is inconclusive, there is still no way to prove the link.

Claims filed by the Bell Cluster employees were rejected by the Workers' Compensation Board. An epidemiologist hired by Bell Canada concluded that the Bell Cluster was random—meaning that the cancer diagnoses were coincidental and not linked to any one thing. Survivors of the Bell Cluster want laws to impose more stringent standards for computer equipment and other sources of electromagnetic radiation, believing it best to err on the side of caution. The Bell Cluster story tells us more about what we don't know and can't prove, but strongly suspect. It illustrates the frustration that cancer prevention advocates face when trying to get an industry to take action to protect workers.

You're more likely to be affected by workplace carcinogens if you work or live in energy-sealed buildings; are exposed to fumes from carpets, pesticides, cleaners, and airborne allergens; are exposed to industrial chemicals, such as those found in plants that process wood, metal, plastics, paints, and textiles; are in constant contact with pesticides, fungicides, and fertilizers; live in high-pollution areas;

and work in dry-cleaning, hair styling, pest control, printing, and photocopying.

This chapter is not about what we don't know and can't prove, rather, it is limited to what we do know and can prove about occupational hazards, as of this writing. One of the problems is that there is a dearth of conclusive scientific evidence to prove cause and effect in the area of occupational carcinogens. For specific information about indoor toxins in the home, see part 1. Radon gas is discussed on page 105. It's important to distinguish between a toxin and a carcinogen. A *toxin* causes a toxic effect (or adverse biological effect). A *carcinogen* causes cancer. A toxin is not the same thing as a carcinogen. Not all toxins cause cancer, and the term *toxic* is not synonymous with *carcinogenic*. And it is important to note that the dose makes the poison. We cannot avoid being exposed to most of the these substances, but the question is: What exposure amount is a concern?

WHAT WE DO KNOW—AND CAN PROVE

In the past, occupational exposure to carcinogens was often severe, and involved direct exposure to carcinogens. In the 1880s, coal miners would inevitably die of lung cancer (known as black lung disease) before the hazard was recognized and controlled through changes in the mining industry and the introduction of protective gear. In areas where we could prove a link between a substance in the workplace and cancer, we got better at removing hazards or protecting workers from those hazards.

For many working North Americans, retirement won't involve more golfing or home decorating; it will involve trips to the hospital for cancer treatment. Occupationally induced cancers will continue to afflict those who entered the workforce before proper controls were introduced. As consumers, we are all affected by industrial hazards since so many of the chemicals in high use have never been tested for human health safety. An arsenal of new chemicals is introduced each year, which puts all of us at risk. In fact, many of the existing chemicals in high use haven't been tested, either.

In a 1999 report on occupational hazards, it was noted that occupational cancers are not evenly distributed throughout the population. Blue-collar workers, such as those in agriculture, mining, metal working, and painting, have five times the rate of occupational cancers. In 1995, Dr. Peter Inante, director of the Office of Standards Review, Occupational Safety, and Health Administration of the U.S. Department of Labor, stated that blue-collar workers "appeared to be the canaries in our society for identifying human chemical carcinogens in the general environment." Nonunionized workers have less access to information on occupational hazards and are also at greater risk. It's also critical to note that other factors also play a role in cancer development, which includes the lifestyle factors discussed in part 1.

Here is what we know so far regarding workplace carcinogens, discussed in alphabetical order:

Agriculture-Related Carcinogens

Concern is growing about the dangers of repeated exposure to herbicides and pesticides. Because of the way food is grown and processed in the West, these chemicals are familiar to just about everyone who shops at the local supermarket. They are of special relevance to people who work in the agricultural industry, such as greenhouse workers, veterinarians, pesticide applicators, pesticide manufacturers, and anyone around pesticides in nonoccupational settings are exposed to these chemicals.

The risk of lymphoma, whereby cancer spreads through the lymph nodes, for example, has increased among agricultural workers. And in Canada, a study of Saskatchewan farmers found a significant association between risk of non-Hodgkin's lymphoma and farmland sprayed with herbicides.

One meta-analysis of twenty different studies spanning eight countries found that compared to the general population, farmers suffer from higher rates of Hodgkin's disease, multiple myeloma, leukemia, skin cancers, and cancers of the lip, stomach, and prostate. A 1999 Swedish study found that four hundred patients with non-Hodgkins lymphoma were 60 percent more likely to report exposure to herbicides and three times more likely to report exposure to fungicides. A later study in 2005 in the journal *Cancer Causes and Control* looked at lymphohematopoietic cancers (LHC) in Hispanic farmworkers in California, concluding that the dangers of pesticides used in agriculture pose a particularly high risk of leukemia among female workers. The study notes that California farmworkers in areas where mancozeb and toxaphene were used had an increased risk of leukemia compared with workers employed elsewhere. Note: Exposure to pesticides and herbicides in home gardening probably does not result in the same risks, because the frequency of exposure is different, and the dose home gardeners are exposed to is different. Home gardeners are not outside everyday spraying one thousand acres or so, which is the case for an agricultural worker. Again, a mantra of toxicology is that the "dose makes the poison."

Asbestos

Asbestos is a naturally occurring mineral that was used to manufacture products such as cement, fireproof textiles, paper, brake linings, vinyl floor tiles, additives for asphalt, resins, plastics, and sealants. It was also used widely for building insulation. Even as early as 1958, industry and government were aware of the health risks associated with asbestos. A 1987 study found a sixfold increase in lung cancer among workers in one plant where asbetsos levels were alarming, whereas families of these workers were being diagnosed with mesothelioma, an asbestos-related lung cancer.

Anyone working in old buildings with asbestos is at a greater risk for a variety of cancers, including lung and gastrointestinal cancers. Severe asbestos exposure, for example, can double the risk of stomach and colorectal cancer, although the cancer can take more than twenty years to develop. Unfortunately, because of the time lapse between exposure and the development of the disease, it is hard to link these cancers to asbestos exposure in any conclusive way, although experts maintain that asbestos can be the cause. Scientific reviews continue to support the notion that none of the various methods used to estimate asbestos exposure yielded consistent trends. Furthermore, the strength of the associations were weak or nonexistent for the four types of gastrointestinal (GI) cancers: stomach, colorectal, colon, and rectal. However, it is well known that asbestos and tobacco make deadly coexposures. Smokers who are exposed to asbestos have a much higher incidence of cancer. Note: Exposure to asbestos in the home results in the same risks.

Dioxin

Dioxin is considered a known human carcinogen and it is associated with higher rates of all kinds of cancers. Although this substance is an environmental estrogen (see chapter 8) a by-product of any chlorinated compound, it is an antiestrogen and blocks the actions of estrogen. In other words, dioxins are not produced intentionally; when chlorinated compounds break down, dioxin is the result. Dioxin, therefore, is a waste product.

Although dioxin is thought to be associated with higher rates of reproductive cancers, it has actually been observed that those exposed to dioxin have a decrease in breast cancer, which is believed to be related to its anti-estrogen effects. Those who work in the platics industry, or who are exposed to bleached paper or incinerators, are exposed to dioxin, but toxicologists insist that a larger dose of dioxin is delivered to an individual who eats fish from contaminated water, or through air pollution.

Secondhand Tobacco Smoke

As we saw in chapter 2, anyone who works in an environment where he or she is exposed to secondhand smoke is at a greater risk for lung cancer and possibly other cancers, such as breast cancer. Some occupational exposures are exacerbated by cigarette smoke, especially asbestos and radon. This complicates matters because it's hard enough to isolate certain carcinogens, but when they attack us in combination, we don't have the scientific measurement techniques in place to track multiple factors appropriately. Note: Exposure to SHS in the home results in the same risks.

Metalworking Fluids

Metalworking fluids (MWF) are the mineral oils, cutting oils, lubricating oils, and coolants used in industries that perform machining, grinding, or forming processes. These substances are linked to an increased risk of cancer of the larynx, rectum, pancreas, skin, scrotum, and bladder. Vegetable-based oils are an alternative lubricant to mineral oils and a number of workplaces are using this substitute. Two studies, both addressing the effects of metalworking fluids on workers in Michigan auto plants, point out their serious risks. One study, in the *American Journal of Industrial Medicine* from 2005, concluded that there is some preliminary evidence for an association between soluble MWF and an increased risk of breast cancer in female autoworkers. Another study, from a 2004 issue of the journal *Occupational and Environmental Medicine*, discovered an association between larynx cancer incidence and MWF exposure.

Methylene Chloride

Methylene chloride is a liquid used in food, furniture, and plastics processing, as well as in paint removing. This substance is labeled as a probable human carcinogen by the U.S. Environmental Protection Agency (EPA) and has been determined to be carcinogenic under the Canadian Environmental Protection Act. Methylene chloride can also cross the placenta and affect fetal development. High levels of methylene chloride are no doubt in all major urban centers across the United States. Fortunately, some states are paying attention to methylene chloride and now routinely monitor it.

Mining Industry–Related Carcinogens

Lung cancers are well-documented examples of occupational exposure to lung carcinogens such as asbestos and radiation in mines. The process involved in nickel refining is also dangerous, although foundry workers, gold miners, and those exposed to chromate are probably at equal risk. For some hard-rock miners, the risk is more pronounced, particularly for nickel and gold miners who were in the workforce prior to 1945. And while it is suspected that the risk in hard-rock miners may in part be due to exposure to radon, there is some evidence that silica may be a carcinogen in its own right. Arsenic, among other culprits, may also have been present.

Perchloroethylene

Known as *perc*, perchloroethylene is the infamous carcinogen associated with dry-cleaning establishments. Perc is used in its vapor or gas form to clean clothes, and has been identified as a probable carcinogen associated with higher rates of cancers of all kinds. Workers in dry-cleaning establishments are at greatest risk, but since so many dry cleaners are located in residential neighborhoods or in multiuse buildings such as apartment complexes, we are all exposed to perc when the vapors are not properly contained. Almost all perc vapors escape into the air. Even when you pick up dry-cleaned clothes, you're exposed to low levels of perc. Perc is also used as a metal degreaser and an ingredient in many chemicals. There is good news to report. New generations of dry-cleaning machines have decreased the release of contaminated air during the loading and unloading processes. A 2006 study in the *Journal of Occupational and Environmental Hygiene* discusses the numbers of workers exposed to perc, and how they have dramatically decreased. Although 25,700 workers in Germany were exposed to perc back in 1975, the number had dropped to below 5,900 since 2001, due in large part to perc being replaced in the industry by nonchlorinated solvents. Individual states are making new laws regarding perc as well. According to the California Air Resources Board

Web site, "Amendments will over time phase out the use of perc dry-cleaning machines and related equipment by January 1, 2023."

Petroleum Industry–Related Carcinogens

There are a number of risks associated with the use or manufacture of petroleum. The following carcinogens are associated with petroleum and other industries:

Benzene

Occupational exposure to benzene, which is a component of gasoline and of some new building adhesives, is thought to cause leukemia. When lead was banned from gasoline, additional benzene was put in some gasoline as an additive. It is also used as a solvent for other petrochemicals such as paint, certain plastics, foams, and pesticides. Workers in the oil and chemical industries are at risk, as well as firefighters, who face benzene exposure as a contaminant in fire smoke.

Consumers are exposed to benzene through tailpipe emissions from cars, and engines found on lawnmowers or leaf-blowers, as well as evaporated gasoline. There are currently no air quality standards in place for benzene.

Diesel Exhaust

Diesel exhaust is considered a probable human carcinogen, and is associated with higher rates of lung cancers in occupational groups exposed to diesel exhaust. Diesel is used in some workplaces to provide electrical power from generators, but the major source of occupational exposure is to public transit workers, taxi and truck drivers, and workers in shipping and handling areas where diesel vehicles idle. The EPA publishes a PDF of state and local anti-idling laws, available at www.epa.gov/region8/air/rmcdc/pdf/CompilationofStateIdlingRegulations.pdf

Polycyclic Aromatic Hydrocarbons

Polycyclic aromatic hydrocarbons (PAHs) are chemicals that are released whenever fuels such as oil, gasoline, coal, and wood are burned. Most of us are exposed to PAHs through emissions from cars, coal-fired generating stations, municipal incinerators, home heating, and industrial furnaces. Particulate matter containing PAHs are often in many air pollutions and can carry PAHs into the lung. Workers in foundries, in aluminum or coke production, in petroleum refining, and workers exposed to asphalt have higher risks of cancer of the esophagus, pancreas, prostate, and lung. A "ToxFAQ" from the U.S. Department of Health and Human Services: Agency for Toxic Substances & Disease Registry, which can be found at www.atsdr.cdc.gov, summarizes that "PAHs may reasonably be expected to be carcinogens. Some people who have breathed or touched mixtures of PAHs and other chemicals for long periods of time have developed cancer. Some PAHs have caused cancer in laboratory animals when they breathed air containing them (lung cancer), ingested them in food (stomach cancer), or had them applied to their skin (skin cancer)." It's hard to isolate PAHs as a single carcinogen because they're always mixed with other substances. PAHs are one of the most potent environmental pollutants.

Carcinogens

Known carcinogens at the office (or home) may be found in the following list, but the one carcinogen that tops the list, outweighing all of the carcinogens below is secondhand smoke:

- Asbestos building materials
- Cleaning products and disinfectants
- Urea-formaldehyde foam insulation
- Adhesives (may contain naphthalene, phenol, cthanol, vinyl chloride, formaldehyde, acrylonitrile, and epoxy, which are toxic substances that release vapors)
- Toners used in copy machines and printers
- Particleboard furniture and space dividers
- Permanent-ink pens and markers (contain acetone, cresol, ethanol, phenol, toluene, and xylene)
- Polystyrene cups
- Synthetic office carpet (may contain acrylic, polyester, and nylon plastic fibers, and formaldehyde-based finishes, pesticides due to mothproofing for wool only)
- Correction fluid (may contain cresol, ethanol, trichloro-ethylene, and naphthalene, which are all toxic chemicals)

Radiation

Radiation is a risk factor for leukemia. We don't yet know how this risk will affect nuclear energy workers. There have been concerns about whether exposure to electromagnetic fields (EMF) might be another cause of leukemia, but the evidence is very weak, and as time goes on, the evidence appears to grow weaker. There is a reputed link between brain tumors and proximity to electromagnetic fields, but this connection is still being investigated, and again, the evidence is weak. Lymphoma is another one of the malignancies that has been linked to exposure to electromagnetic fields, but nuclear energy workers did not show a significant association with lymphoma in studies done to date, and the evidence remains weak. A 2006 review article in the journal *Cancer Causes and Control* also suggests that overall the evidence available to date does not suggest an increased risk of breast cancer related to EMF exposure. Nor is there conclusive proof of EMF causing the Bell Cluster cancers, discussed at the beginning of this chapter.

The massive proliferation of cell phone usage around the world in the last few years may beg the question, what kinds of cancer risks exist with increased human exposure to radiofrequency (RF) fields? The evidence is weak in the correlation between cancer and RFs. The National Cancer Institute is following this issue closely at: www.cancer.gov/cancertopics/factsheet/Risk/cellphones.

For More Information

Specific concerns can be explored through the NIOSH-TIC database, maintained by the U.S. National Institute of Occupational Safety and Health (NIOSH). In Canada, the Canadian Centre for Occupational Health and Safety, www.ccohs.ca, provides plenty of information on workplace environments and safety issues.

126

HOW DO WE PROTECT OURSELVES FROM WORKPLACE CARCINOGENS?

Since so many environmental carcinogens originate in the workplace, and are then emitted into the air, water, or land, eliminating carcinogens in the workplace—at the source—would have a huge impact on cleaning up the environment in general. The National Institute of Environmental Health Sciences (NIEHS), which can be found at www.niehs.nih.gov, is working on personal biosensors that can be used to monitor an individual's exposure.

A woefully inadequate body of knowledge exists about workplace carcinogens. In urban centers, residents are exposed to a wide array of carcinogens in their workplaces, but there is only clear evidence of the cancer-causing potential for nine substances (known as the "noxious nine"): benzene, diesel exhaust, polycyclic aromatic hydrocarbons, perchloroethylene, dioxin, pesticides, metalworking fluids, methylene chloride, and asbestos.

As for the rest of the long list of suspected carcinogens, researchers point to the need for more research in the future. The most important investigation into workplace carcinogens is the ongoing review process at the International Agency for Research on Cancer (IARC), whose mission is to "coordinate and conduct research on the causes of human cancer, the mechanisms of carcinogenesis, and to develop scientific strategies for cancer control." (See the Web site www.iarc.fr.)

The absence of information or conclusive proof is not the same thing as the absence of risk. Many cancer experts assert that the goal of industry ought to be zero risk in the workplace by taking a precautionary or "seat belt" approach; currently, we settle for an "acceptable risk." For instance, wearing a seat belt in a car is a precautionary approach; we don't know for sure if we'll have an accident, but we have enough evidence to know that we must be careful on the roads. Similarly, we can prevent the risk of carcinogen exposure by not allowing untested substances to be used until proven safe.

By now, you'd think that we could simply ban known workplace carcinogens and use our scientific knowledge to find substitutes. Sometimes the only way to do this is to ban the worker instead of the substance. If a carcinogenic substance is essential to the manufacturing process, protective clothing and other equipment, as well as improved ventilation systems (such as those used in the mining industry), are ways to control exposure.

Thus, carcinogenic exposure in the workplace has been reduced to the extent where it can no longer be proven that workers are at any greater risk than the general public. This is the case, for example, with hard-rock miners. It does seem plausible, in such circumstances, that those who joined the workforce in the last few years are at no greater risk of occupationally induced cancers than the rest of us.

Government's Response

What protections are in place for workers when it comes to workplace carcinogens? Governments have long recognized their obligation to introduce regulations to reduce or, if possible, prevent exposure to carcinogens in the workplace. In lieu of measures that would guarantee zero exposure, governments have recognized that it is up to them to compensate for cancer caused by occupational exposure. Most workers' compensation boards do just that, using a set of guidelines to evaluate the relative toxicity of certain established carcinogens. What we need to do is establish that suspected carcinogenic chemicals are dangerous from the outset. Workers' right-to-know legislation exists in several states and provinces, which ought to identify hazardous chemicals and material safety information. But experts are concerned that right-to-know documents cover too few substances; for example, effluents or by-products and all pesticides are frequently exempt. The state of California has been a leader in providing timely chemical information to workers and employers, as well as the public, through a program known as Cal/OSHA, and the Hazard Evaluation System and Information Service.

Hazards, such as 9/11

We live in a scary post-9/11 world where bioterrorism is a real threat. Workers in New York City were exposed to dangerous toxins as a result of the terrorist attack on the World Trade Center (WTC) on September 11, 2001. This created an environmental disaster within the confines of a small geographic area. The populations at greatest risk for exposure to the toxins in the air (pulverized cement, glass, asbestos, lead, dioxins, and cement dust, to name a few) were the first responders on the scene: firefighters, police, and paramedics. Also at risk were community residents, especially women who were pregnant on that day, as well as those who took part in the cleanup in the area at surrounding buildings and on the streets. An early study in a 2004 paper in the journal *Environmental Health Perspectives*, which is one of the earliest detailed studies of the disaster, hypothesizes about some of the potential for cancer to arise in those exposed to dioxin in the days following the attack. At that time it was an unknown risk. Most papers on the topic focus on the enormity of respiratory illnesses, including the "World Trade Center cough" that came about from exposure.

By the 10th anniversary, a plethora of new studies and papers have been released about the environmental health effects associated with the World Trade Center collapse. The most documented risks involve respiratory health problems and the risk of lung cancers, including mesothelioma. There are still questions about other cancers directly related to 9/11 dust, but many of those exposed are developing cancers at higher rates than in the general population.

After years of delays, Congress finally passed the James Zadroga 9/11 Health Compensation Act, which was signed into law in 2011. And in 2012, 58 cancers directly related to 9/11 exposures were added to the list of 9/11 health conditions for which the Act is designed to compensate. For more information, visit: http://www.nyc.gov/html/doh/wtc/html/health_compensation/health_compensation_act.shtml

TESTING FOR TOXICITY

Testing for toxicity means proving that something is poisonous. This is often done by exposing a rat to a substance and seeing if the rat gets sick or dies. Researchers measure the dose of poison that causes illness or death. This is much easier to prove than trying to establish whether a particular poisonous substance causes cancer.

All industrialized countries share information about workplace hazards and toxic chemicals. It's no surprise that the United States is the yardstick by which Canadians measure their knowledge base—and Canada is only as safe from industrial carcinogens as its American cousin. So, how is the United States faring when it comes to knowledge about occupational hazards? The sad truth is not very well at all. There are, we must keep in mind, organizations such Environmental Defense, founded by scientists over forty years ago, which strive to educate the public by "partnering with businesses, governments and communities to find practical environmental solution." (See www.environmentaldefense.org.) Their scientific research, for example, led to safer drinking water standards via the Safe Drinking Water Act of 1974.

There is a perception among the American public that because of knowledge regarding dangerous chemicals such as DDT, lead, and PCBs, there is much more safety and knowledge in the workplace regarding chemical carcinogens. The U.S. Congress even passed the Toxic Substances Control Act more than twenty years ago. Yet, according to the latest data from the U.S. Environmental Defense Fund, for most of the important chemicals in U.S. commerce, the simplest safety facts still don't exist. Even in this new century, the most basic toxicity testing results don't exist in the public record for nearly 75 percent of the top-volume chemicals in commercial use.

In the early 1980s, the U.S. National Academy of Sciences' National Research Council completed a four-year study revealing that 78 percent of the chemicals in high-volume use had not been tested. When you consider that nearly 71 percent of the tested chemicals in high-volume use do not pass health hazard screening set by the Organization for Economic Cooperation and Development (OECD) Chemicals Program, this fact becomes all the more frightening. But we were still living in ignorance about what chemical harms may or may not be in the environment as late as the mid-1990s. In its recent report, the U.S. Environmental Defense Fund stated: "Guinea pig status is not what Congress promised the public more than twenty years ago.

Instead, it established a national policy that the risks of toxic chemicals in our environment would be identified and controlled. Ignorance, pervasive and persistent over the course of twenty years, has made that promise meaningless." (Environmental Defense Fund Report, 1997:6)

Getting Industry on Board

As consumers, we must remind industry that we want to know the safety biographies of the products we're buying. All chemicals in high-volume use in North America ought to have been screened for at least preliminary health effects with the results publicly available for verification. A model definition of what should be included in preliminary screening tests for high-volume chemicals was developed and agreed on in 1990 by the United States and the other member nations of the OECD, which includes Canada. All we've been waiting for is the industry's commitment to let the screenings begin. As consumers, we can boycott products that don't give us information about manufacturing safety, which we deserve.

We already know what we don't know about industry chemicals. So the first step in protecting our workers—and ourselves—is finding out more by demanding "hazard identification," which means doing screening tests for health safety chemical by chemical. Obviously, not all chemicals are toxic, but we ought to know which ones are. Here's what we should demand from any industry using chemicals:

- *Toxicity screening.* These are pretty easy tests that can tell us how toxic a chemical is, and what forms of toxicity are involved. This is different from testing for cancer-causing potential. The challenge is that it's not that simple to determine if a chemical is poisonous and "not good for us" without clear goals for what to measure. A major problem is that for cancer, there is a twenty-year lag period on average between exposure and diagnosis. In addition, since lifestyle plays a role, it may make sense to ultimately identify who may be most susceptible to chemical X or Y, as the more important goal. In 1998, the U.S. EPA reported that there is no basic toxicity screening for 43 percent of the three thousand chemicals used in the United States in quantities of one million pounds per year or more. Only 7 percent of these three thousand chemicals have a full set of basic test data. The EPA estimated in 1998 that it would cost only 0.2 percent of the total annual sales of the top U.S. chemical companies to fill all of the basic screening data gaps for high-production volume chemicals.

- *Answers to the following about each chemical after screening.* It's not enough for an industry to say, "Yep, we tested this chemical and it's safe." The following questions are based on internationally accepted criteria for toxicity screening created by the OECD Chemicals Program in 1990. If we know the answers to the following, we will know a toxic chemical's potential to be a human health hazard.

  » What happens when you're exposed one time to chemical X (known as acute toxicity)?
  » What happens when you're exposed continuously to chemical X (known as repeated dose toxicity)?
  » What happens to a fetus's genes if a pregnant woman is exposed to chemical X (known as in vitro genetic toxicity)?
  » What happens to your own body or genes when you're exposed to chemical X (known as in vivo genetic toxicity)?
  » What happens to your reproductive organs (ovaries, breasts, breast milk, or testicles) when exposed to chemical X?
  » What happens to a developing fetus (limbs, brain, etc.) when exposed to chemical X (known as developmental toxicity/teratogenicity)?

- *The "next steps" for each chemical tested.* We should know which chemicals require no further testing, which chemicals require more testing, and which chemicals need to be controlled.
- *Open-door policies on chemical information.* In chapter 2, we saw that for years the tobacco industry has been guilty of hiding its research on the dangers of tobacco from the public. We want assurance that this is not going on in other industries, and we should demand that all private tests on specific chemicals that major manufacturers have performed or paid for—which to date have not been made available to the public—be made available to us. Trade secrets about a chemical should only be maintained long enough for appropriate testing to be conducted. After that, information about the chemical should be made public if it affects the public.
- *A ban on all "high-production-volume chemicals" that haven't been*

tested. Any chemical currently produced or imported in quantities of more than one million pounds per year should not be allowed to be in use without toxicity testing. For example, we don't know how 53 percent of high-priority chemicals affect our reproductive organs, whether 63 percent of high-priority chemicals cause cancer, whether 67 percent of high-priority chemicals affect our nervous systems or brain function, whether 86 percent of high-priority chemicals affect our immune systems, and how 90 percent of high-priority chemicals affect our children's health.

Getting Government on Board

As consumers, we should demand from our federal and state/provincial governments nothing less than what the Environmental Defense Fund demands in the face of ignorance. To get the ball rolling, write to your federal and state departments/provincial ministries of labor and environment and demand the following:

- Ask for government incentives to industry to gather and disclose screening information about major chemicals and to take early steps to reduce the use of, and prevent exposures to, chemicals that have been identified as hazardous or that have not been screened. Clearly, so much depends on who is in power in the White House, for example. As a 2007 AP press release notes: "The White House pressured the Environmental Protection Agency to weaken requirements that companies annually disclose releases of toxic chemicals . . . the changes mean that industry will have to file 22,000 fewer reports each year, reducing an important public monitoring tool on industrial emissions."

- Demand that public disclosure on all tested chemicals be made available, and appropriately identified as *safe, potentially safe* (this means they are presumed safe but not absolutely proven to be safe), *harmful,* or *potentially harmful* (meaning that they are presumed harmful but not absolutely proven to be harmful). The EPA does provide up-to-date access to NESHAP: The National Emission Standards for Hazardous Air Pollutants, most recently updated in January 2008, via its publicly available site: www.epa.gov/ttn/atw/mactfnlalph.html. NESHAP even gives compliance dates, so that consumers can see when the standard came into effect.

133

- Demand that public disclosure on all untested chemicals be made available. A separate database should be created that lists all untested chemicals with a designation of "unknown risks" attached. Chemicals entered on this database should be given priority according to high-volume usage (over a million pounds per year), so the chemicals used most get listed first until, eventually, all untested chemicals are listed.

- Demand a ban on any new, untested chemicals from entering the environment. Nothing new and untested should be used in industry until the old, untested chemicals have been tested properly. Then new chemicals can be introduced only after they've passed testing requirements. The suggestion for mutagenicity testing for new chemicals has been made in some regions. This is a red-flag test that tells us whether further testing for carcinogenicity is needed.

- Demand that the medical community begin compiling detailed work histories on all cancer patients so that patterns of exposure can be linked with certain cancers. This is valuable information that we currently don't have.

Nobody knows whether or not a large majority of the highest-use chemicals are under control. We really don't know what we're likely to breathe or drink or house in our bodies. And we don't know what is being released from industrial facilities into our backyards, streets, forests, and streams.

A lot of what you've read in this chapter has likely disturbed you. In the book, *Exposed: The Toxic Chemistry of Everyday Products and What's at Stake for American Power*, author Mark Shapiro, discusses the differences between hazardous substances monitoring in the European Union and the United States. "Since 2004, the EU has banned entire categories of hazardous chemicals from use in cosmetics, toys, electronics, and other consumer goods." This latest EU regulation, known as REACH, "is a new European Community Regulation on chemicals and their safe use (EC 1907/2006). It deals with the **R**egistration, **E**valuation, **A**uthorization, and restriction of **CH**emical substances. The new law entered into force on June 1 2007." (See, http://ec.europa.eu/environment/chemicals/reach/reach_intro.htm.)

Perhaps the most impressive aspect of REACH is the great responsibility it places on industry to manage the dangers of chemicals, and to also provide consistent and understandable safety information on the substances in question. This is something for the whole world to aspire to.

The "Least-Wanted List" of Known Cancer Agents

There is sufficient evidence to prove these substances cause cancer in humans. This is a partial list.

Chemical	Type of Cancer
Acrylonitrile	Lung
4-Aminobiphenyl	Urinary bladder
Arsenic	Lung, skin
Asbestos	Lung, several others
Benzene	Leukemia (white blood cells)
Benzidine	Urinary bladder
Beryllium	Lung
Bis-chloromethyl ether (BCME)	Lung
Chloromethyl methyl ether	Lung
Chromates, most types	Lung, larynx, nasal cavity
Coal Tar	Lung, skin, bladder
Ethylene oxide	Lymphatic, blood
Metalworking fluids	Skin, larynx, rectum, stomach, esophagus, colon, bladder, sinonasal, lung, prostate, pancreas
Mustard gas	Lung
2-Naphthylamine	Urinary bladder
Nickel and its compounds	Lung, nasal cavity
Polycyclic aromatic hydrocarbons	Lung, several others
(PAHs), poly nuclera aromatics, (PNAs)—includes coke oven emissions, soot, and various kinds of smoke), radon	Lung
Tobacco smoke—secondhand smokers	Lung, mouth, larynx, lips, throat, bladder, kidney, pancreas
Vinyl chloride	Liver, brain, lymphatic, blood
Wood dusts (limited types)	Nasal cavity, possibly others

Chemicals Under Suspicion

Many chemicals are under suspicion because they have been proven to cause cancer in animals but have not yet been conclusively shown to cause human cancer. The list is long. Here are some of the more common ones:

Cadmium
Carbon tetrachloride
Chloroform
Dibromochlorpropane (DBCP)
Diesel exhaust
Ethylene theourea
Formaldehyde
Isocyanates
Kepone
MOCA (aka curene or methylene-bis-chloroaniline)
Nitrosamines
PCBs (poly chlorinated biphenyls)
Perchloroethylene ("perc")
Trichloroethylene (TCE)
Tris 2, 3 dibromoppropyl phosphate ("Tris")
Vinyl bromide

Source: The Canadian Autoworkers Health and Safety Department. Cancer in Your Workplace: A Manual for Worker Investigators. 1999:28–29.

Scenes of the Crime

Possible high-risk jobs: These jobs can involve exposure to known animal or human carcinogens.

Job	Carcinogen
Brake-shoe manufacture	Asbestos
Pipefitting	Asbestos
Selected welding and grinding jobs	Beryllium, chromium, cadmium, nickel, stainless steel (chrome and nickel)
Forming and curing certain plastics	Acrylonitrile, MOCA (aka curene or methylene-bis-chloroaniline), formaldehyde, styrene

Job	Carcinogen
Degreasing and cold cleaning with chlorinated solvents	Trichloroethylene
Foundry core-making	Formaldehyde
Metalworking engine plants, metalworking fluids components plants, parts plants, aerospace, machine shops, mining, smelting, and milling	Diesel exhaust, oil mists, radon gas, arsenic, PAHs, EMFs (electro magnetic fields)

Source: *The Canadian Autoworkers Health and Safety Department.* Cancer in Your Workplace: A Manual for Worker Investigators. *1999:30*

Workplaces under Investigation

These workplaces are under suspicion because of preliminary cancer studies. More work is needed to pin down specific jobs or chemicals.

- Foundry work, especially core-making and exposure to mold burn-off
- Machining operations with oil and coolant mist (e.g., bearing plants, engine plants)
- Wood model and pattern making
- Motor vehicle assembly plants
- Plating and die-casting operations
- Smelters—PAHs, EMFs, nickel

Jobs with Special Considerations

- *Processes with oil smoke, such as forging operations, heat treat, or hot die work.* Many of these jobs involve exposure to various polycyclic aromatic hydrocarbons (PAHs), some of which are known to cause human cancer. Adequate air measurements or mortality studies have not been done in most cases.
- *Work around diesel exhaust.* Diesel particulate can carry various PAH chemicals deep into the lung. It is known that diesel exhaust can cause serious damage to bacteria. Excess cancers have been seen among locomotive engineers and miners.
- *Fiberglass fabrication.* Dust from small-diameter fiberglass is a cancer hazard, depending on the size and shape of the glass fiber.

137

- *Work with metalworking fluids.* Scientific studies have shown that workers in a variety of industries are at high cancer risk. The specific types of cancer vary and the chemicals responsible are not fully established in all cases:

Job	Carcinogen
Rubber industry workers	Nitrosamines, NDMA (nitrosodimethylamine)
Uranium miners	Radon gas
Nickel smelting workers	Nickel
Petroleum refinery workers	Benzene
Aluminum smelting workers	EMFs, PAHs
Copper smelting workers	Arsenic
Roofers	Coal tar, PAHs
Hematite miners, leather and shoe workers	Chromates
Printing press workers	Solvents
Hospital operating room personnel	Ethylene oxide
Wood products workers	Pentachlorophenol, creosote, arsenic, chromium (wood preservatives)
Chemical dye manufacturers	Benzidines

Source: The Canadian Autoworkers Health and Safety Department. Cancer in Your Workplace: A Manual for Worker Investigators. 1999:31.

CHAPTER 9

EARTH, WIND, AND FIRE

One of the most unsettling experiences of my life came a number of years ago while watching a *Sesame Street* vignette called, "Where Does Rain Come From?" As my then four-year-old niece sat with her apple juice, fascinated by the story of clouds, air condensation, and all the other interesting facts behind what makes rain, all I could think of was how interconnected everything was, and how airborne contaminants could easily poison our water, and vice versa. If you know where rain comes from, you know how dangerous airborne contaminants are to our health. By taking a closer look at the accumulation of toxic substances in our air, water, and food supply, we can begin to explore what has been increasingly recognized as a major threat to human health.

ENVIRONMENTAL CARCINOGENS

In 1962, environmentalist Rachel Carson wrote a book called *Silent Spring*, which essentially said to wake up and smell the chemicals because wildlife and humans are dying from exposure to pesticides and pollutants. Carson was denounced by industry and medical leaders as hysterical; she died of breast cancer in 1964. Today, many renowned scientists in both the environmental and medical research community are concluding that maverick Rachel Carson was right all along. In the mid-1990s, two next-generation *Silent Spring* texts were published. Dr. Theo Colborne, a senior scientist at the World Wildlife Fund and co-author of *Our Stolen Future* (1996), and Dr. Sandra Steingraber, author of *Living Downstream: An Ecologist Looks at Cancer and The Environment* (1997), were hailed as the voice of primary prevention cancer advocates who took on Rachel Carson's cause. Dr. Steingraber put it best at a lecture she gave in 1997 at the World Conference on Breast Cancer: "Science likes to prove the same thing over and over again before it says that something is fact. And that's usually a good thing. But sometimes calling for more research is the grandfather excuse for doing nothing." This sentiment is echoed by the International Joint Commission on the Great Lakes:

> Scientific arguments and their lack of absolute proof can also be used as an excuse for inaction. The phrase "good science" has been used to block change through demands for more rigorous proof. (*Eighth Biennial Report On Great Lakes Water Quality*, 1996, p. 17).

The term *environmental carcinogens* refers to cancer-causing agents that are in our environment: the air, soil, and water. So whatever comes into contact with this air, soil and water can become contaminated. The implications for our food chain are clear—plants and animals nourished by contaminated soil and water become contaminated.

A list of persistent toxic substances put together by the Accelerated Reduction/Elimination of Toxins (ARET) project, contained more than seventy identified or suspected carcinogens in the air we breathe or the water we drink. Carcinogens on ARET's A-1 list (those that met or exceeded ARET's criteria for toxicity, accumulation, and persistence) include all polychlorinated biphenyls; polycyclic aromatic hydrocarbons (PAHs); 1,8-dinitro-pyrene; and five types of chlorinated organics, also called organochlorines. The substances on all these lists are in the air, the soil, and the water around us. See the IARC tables at the end of this chapter for a complete list (or what we know so far).

What Are We Breathing?

We are exposed to countless known or suspected carcinogens every day. Present in our air, our water, our soil, and consequently our food, these contaminants are impossible to avoid. Our skin absorbs them, our lungs inhale them, and we ingest them just about every time we eat.

A two-year study in Windsor, Ontario—which is near Detroit, Michigan—was undertaken in response to concerns that air pollution was drifting across the Canada-U.S. border. The community was worried about the quality of both outdoor and indoor air—and for good reason. Forty air pollutants were investigated, ten of which have been known to cause risks to human health in the long term. Five of these ten pollutants were found to be present in high concentrations in both indoor and outdoor air. Benzene, 1,3-butadiene, and chromium (VI) raised cancer risks via indoor and outdoor air; while cadmium, carbon tetrachloride, 1,4-dichlorobenzene, formaldehyde, and PAHs increased cancer risk via indoor air. Air pollution from coal-burning plants, for example, is associated with major health and environmental impacts. Sadly, as the Ohio Environmental Council points out on its Web site www.theoec.org, "None of Ohio's coal-burning power plants are currently required to follow the strict emissions standards of the Clear Air Act of 1970." This, despite the fact the Ohio ranks number one for both soot and acid rain causing sulfur dioxide, and for smog-causing nitrogen oxide. There is available technology to not only have power plants reduce harmful emissions by over 90 percent but also to "keep the lights on."

Car Exhaust

Car exhaust (known as *vehicle emissions*) is considered to be among the primary sources of carcinogens in the air supply of many Western countries. Car exhaust powered by fossil fuels contains a number of suspected carcinogens, including benzene and polycyclic aromatic hydrocarbons.

What Are We Ingesting?

The most serious hazards affecting our food are what are called *persistent toxic substances*. These are so named because they are, well, *persistent*. They remain in the biophysical environment for long periods of time and become widely dispersed, establishing themselves in the plants, animals, and humans that ingest them as part of the food chain. Sadly, the ecosystem is incapable of breaking down many of these substances. Because they are not naturally occurring chemicals (with their own built-in metabolic pathways for detoxifying themselves), the ecosystem has no way to absorb them. In fact, many of these chemicals have been developed *because* they are not readily metabolized and detoxified. They stick around and, by so doing, cause any number of adverse health effects, including cancer in humans and animals.

We can be pretty certain that persistent toxic substances in our water and soil have entered our food chain. A 2007 review paper on mycotoxins ("secondary fungal metabolites") in the food chain, published in the *Asia Pacific Journal of Clinical Nutrition*, noted that cancer is one of the chronic conditions that has higher incidence following continual exposure to mycotoxin ingestion, particularly in vulnerable, developing countries. According to the review paper, "It has been estimated that 25 percent of the world's crops are affected by mold or fungal growth." Even in North America, toxic chemicals abound in places like the Great Lakes Basin, prompting successive reports by the International Joint Commission. The *Twelfth Biennial Report in 2004* projects into the future: "Site-specific advisories continue to limit or ban consumption of certain fish caught in the Great Lakes because of methyl mercury contamination. In fact, due to localized contaminated sediment, methyl mercury–related fish consumption advisories are expected to last for decades to come in some Great Lakes Areas of Concern" (p. 39). The fact that these substances are being absorbed into our food chain is cause for alarm. It is one of the most compelling reasons we have for sunsetting (meaning, "ridding within a certain timetable") persistent toxic substances that are known or suspected carcinogens.

Organochlorines

Certain classes of persistent toxic chemicals are particularly dangerous. To curtail the risks associated with them, it may make sense to deal with these chemicals as a class or group, instead of addressing them one at a time. Organochlorines are a case in point.

Organochlorines make up a class of chemicals created by the combination of chlorine and various organic compounds, including chemicals such as DDT, PCBs, dioxin, chlordane, and hexachlorobenzene. Many of these substances are also considered animal carcinogens and are thought to be possible human carcinogens. Some organochlorines can impair our immune systems or mimic estrogen and, most serious of all, cause our bodies to grow tumors.

Organochlorines get into the soil, giving them a direct route into the food chain—which is how they get into human beings. Trace residues of organochlorines have shown up in the fatty tissues of birds, animals, and humans. They have also been found in human breast milk. Thankfully, some chlorinated organics, including PCBs and DDT, have been banned, but others continue to be used in pesticides. Organochlorines are also used in the making of polyvinyl chloride (PVC) plastics, and are produced in the bleaching process at pulp and paper mills and the incineration process of chlorine-containing products, such as yogurt containers and plastic bags.

Radioactivity

Our collective fears around radiation exposure have escalated in recent years following events such as the Chernobyl nuclear accident in 1986. Exposure to hazardous levels of radiation has long been recognized as a cause of leukemia and other cancers, particularly thyroid cancer, as a result of radioactive iodine, a substance that is emitted in the fallout caused by nuclear explosions.

To date, the Chernobyl accident was still the most dangerous due to the location of the disaster, which was not on the ocean, like Japan's nuclear reactors (Japan's nuclear reactors suffered a meltdown after the 2011 earthquake/

tsunami disaster). The Chernobyl accident in the former Soviet Union released 40 million curies of radioactive iodine into the atmosphere, exposing millions of people to excessive levels of radioactive iodine. People living within 30 kilometers (18.6 miles) of the accident inhaled the radioactive iodine, and people living outside this radius were exposed to the substance. The incidence of thyroid cancer in children in Belarus, Russia, and the Ukraine appears to have increased twentyfold as a result of exposure. In a report called "Chernobyl's Legacy: Health, Environment, and Sociological Impacts," produced by the Chernobyl Forum and summarized in a WHO press release. The report looks back at the twenty-year impact of this environmental disaster, stating that there were four thousand cases of thyroid cancer, mainly in children at the time of the accident, with the survival rate, fortunately, being almost 99 percent. Furthermore, they estimate the total number of deaths connected to Chernobyl to be about 4,000, with some 3,900 of those being from radiation-induced cancer and leukemia. Oddly, and unexpectedly, nature and wildlife is now thriving in the human-deserted contaminated areas of Chernobyl, raising questions about what the long-term effects truly are regarding nuclear disaster areas. In the United States, a 2006 paper in the journal *Epidemiology* looked at thyroid disease associated with exposure to the Nevada nuclear weapons test site radiation. The paper concluded, "Persons exposed to radioactive iodine as children have an increased risk of thyroid neoplasms and autoimmune thyroiditis up to 30 years after exposure."

The North Dakota State Health Department reported in 1994 that the incidence of thyroid cancer in that state had doubled from 5 percent to 10 percent, an increase that was attributed to radioactive iodine fallout. Furthermore, the U.S. Energy Research Foundation concludes that there may be thousands of North Americans who ingested milk contaminated by this fallout, and who are at greater risk for thyroid cancer. The Oak Ridge Health Agreement Steering Panel reports that of women born in 1952, those in the midwestern United States who drank milk contaminated by the test fallout are more likely to develop thyroid cancer in their lifetime than are women who were born in the northeastern states.

Evidence has been collected from the studies of people with medical exposures to high doses of radiation, and from the studies of atomic bomb survivors in Japan, which indicates that the improper management, storage, and disposal of nuclear waste can produce harmful effects (i.e., cancer) in people who live and work close to the waste products.

Tritium

Tritium, a radioactive isotope of hydrogen, is a by-product of nuclear reactor operations. It cannot be removed from drinking water with conventional water treatment systems. The EPA in the United States classifies tritium as a human carcinogen. Some monitoring of tritium is occurring, with one example being in California. A 2006 government report from the California Office of Environmental Health Hazard Assessment noted that the state has "monitored drinking water supply wells from 1994 to 2001 for various radioactive contaminants including tritium. Tritium was not found to exceed the MCL of 20,000 pCi/L at any source during that period."

HOW DO WE KNOW THESE SUBSTANCES ARE DANGEROUS?

We know what we're breathing and ingesting is probably dangerous based on an accumulating body of scientific evidence, which includes:

- Studies, such as those done on the emission of diesel exhaust, that have identified air pollution as a cause of lung cancer. Other studies have found high rates of lung cancer among people living near large petrochemical plants. One study identified a link between sulfur dioxide and ground-level ozone emissions with the incidence of breast and colon cancers.
- Ecological studies, such as those that prove proximity to a hazardous waste site can increase the risk of breast and other cancers.
- Studies conducted on animals that show a positive correlation between organochlorines and breast cancer. A possible link also exists between breast cancer and exposure to xenoestrogens, estrogen-like substances released into the environment as pesticides or industrial chemicals, which accumulate in body fat. The more estrogen women are exposed to in their lifetime, the greater their risk of breast cancer. However, evidence of the association between organochlorines (often made up of xenoestrogens) and breast cancer is inconclusive.
- Studies that identify exposure to hazardous levels of radiation as a cause of leukemia. There is also a suspected association between leukemia and exposure to electromagnetic fields.
- Results of a metanalysis (a review of other studies) that demonstrated the danger of water disinfection by-products such as chlorinated

organics (formed when chlorine meets naturally occurring humic and fulvic acids). These toxins may be responsible for some ten thousand bladder and rectal cancer deaths in the United States each year.

Limitations of Science

As stated earlier, the problem with proving that all of these environmental hazards are affecting our health is that we can't prove it beyond a reasonable doubt. We suspect but can't absolutely prove, which is why it's so hard to get government and industry to take action to eliminate environmental contaminants. Showing that a substance is toxic is different from linking that toxic substance to negative human health effects. Business and government like to act based on conclusive evidence provided by science. We will never be able to provide that proof because *science* is still unsure about certain untested or poorly tested environmental contaminants. What can we do? If we want to protect our health, we need to demand that the government should never assume that a chemical is safe until it is proven to be safe. Why is the science so unreliable? There are limits to the scientific methods used to do these studies. There's no way to control a study looking at the effects of environmental toxins on human health because:

- *There are too many variables.* We are exposed to a wide variety of environmental pollutants every day. Often, it is a combination of many substances that creates risk, which may also have to do with our genetic makeup. These combinations vary according to where we live, our economic status, our lifestyle, and our work. Trying to figure out which parts of each combination of exposures are attributable to pollution in the environment can be very difficult.
- *We can't "control" whole populations for a study.* For many substances, especially those that have been widely dispersed in the environment, control groups (those that haven't been exposed and can, therefore, act as a point of reference) are impossible to find. It's also difficult to find and assess groups of people with different levels of exposure because these substances are everywhere. Most human populations, for example, now carry detectable levels of suspected carcinogens (e.g., DDT, PCBs) in their body fat.

- *We need to study things for a long time.* The length of time required for accurate results hinders our attempts to put numbers to the cancer/pollution association. Often, only small groups of people have experienced high levels of exposure. Or, we must wait years to confirm a cancer diagnosis. Sometimes, too, subjects withdraw from a study, or the study is abandoned due to high costs.

- *There are too many toxins to study.* We have yet to accumulate toxicological data on some 80 percent of the 45,000 to 100,000 chemicals in common use today. Data on chronic effects are especially limited. However, more than 1,000 chemicals (or combinations of chemicals) have been evaluated by the IARC (see the material at the end of this chapter), and only 30 of them have been found to be carcinogenic. Another 20 are classified as probably carcinogenic to humans and 93 as possibly carcinogenic. It is important to remember that much evidence is needed to identify a substance as carcinogenic. Many chemicals have been identified as "probable" or "possible" carcinogens simply because we lack the proof to call them "known." On the brighter side, many substances are selected for assessment by the IARC based on preliminary evidence that they are carcinogenic; this evidence is only suggestive. Many of the untested substances may not be carcinogenic at all.

- *Existing data is still being attacked.* Not all scientists agree with the studies to date, and many insist they are not proof of anything. Interpretations of data differ for a number of reasons: the dose-level administered in animal testing is often inconsistent; it's difficult to draw conclusions for one species based on the results from testing on another, completely different species; and the models used and assumptions made during testing often don't translate into human risk factor at the other end of the process. The bottom line is that the "solid proof" model is unworkable when dealing with environmental carcinogens and should be abandoned in favor of new approaches outlined next.

The Weight of Evidence Approach

Since we have yet to see any real proof as defined by conventional science of the health risks caused by environmental toxins, we need to work with what we have. That means adopting a "weight of evidence" approach to assessing risk, combining results from different fields of study, including wildlife observations and laboratory testing. That doesn't mean we should halt future research; rather, we shouldn't wait for any further research before beginning to act on what we know now. For instance, estimates of the proportion of cancers caused by environmental carcinogens vary from 2 to 20 percent. It's hard to come up with exact numbers since most of them are based on a combination of daily and workplace exposures. As consumers, we should be informed by science, but our governments have a responsibility to be informed of our values as consumers and citizens, which means they must err on the side of caution.

WHAT ARE THE HEALTH RISKS?

In her book *Living Downstream*, Dr. Sandra Steingraber notes that beluga whales in the polluted St. Lawrence River have high rates of bladder, stomach, intestinal, salivary gland, breast, and ovarian cancers. Meanwhile, beluga whales in the Atlantic Ocean are cancer-free. Steingraber herself was diagnosed with bladder cancer at the age of 20. She quotes conservationist Leone Pippard:

> Tell me, does the St. Lawrence beluga drink too much alcohol and does the St. Lawrence beluga smoke too much and does the St. Lawrence beluga have a bad diet? Is that why the beluga whales are ill? Do you think you are somehow immune and that it's only the beluga whale that is being affected? (Steingraber, Sandra. *Living Downstream*. Addison-Wesley, 1997:139.)

Persistent bioconcentrating toxic substances, meaning toxic substances that live in human and animal fat or settle onto plants, have been linked to all manner of disease and disorder in humans and animals. These toxins can affect everything from reproductive health and immune system functions to behavior and respiratory systems. For example, ground-level ozone, which forms when car exhaust and industry gases interact with the sunlight, is known to cause decreased lung capabilities and other respiratory problems.

Some of the most disturbing evidence documenting the harmful effects of environmental pollutants comes from wildlife studies conducted in areas close to heavy industrial activity. Wildlife exposed to industrial chemicals, for example, show abnormally high numbers of birth defects and reproductive disorders. This phenomenon is almost certainly caused by a sort of "confusion" of natural, biological processes. Environmental contaminants in this case mimic the effect of naturally occurring hormones, disrupting the animal's natural life functions.

Endrocrine Disruptors

Environmental scientists began to notice that several wildlife species are experiencing hermaphroditic traits. In Florida's swamplands, alligators were simply not breeding. A concerned research team from the University of Florida went into the swamps to find out why. These researchers pulled male alligators out of the water to examine their genitals. The majority of male alligators they found were sterile as a result of either nondeveloped or abnormally shaped penises. A chemical spill in nearby waters was found to be the culprit, which was having an "estrogenic effect" on the alligators' natural habitat.

A 2007 study, in the journal *Environmental Health Perspectives*, considers the health impacts of estrogens in the environment, focusing specifically on wastewater treatment effluents as the main cause of reproductive disruption in wild fish populations. The data revealed a strong link between estrogens present in effluents and varied adverse, sex-related problems.

Researchers in Sweden and the United Kingdom have been concerned since the late 1980s over a dramatic increase in male infertility in their countries, while there is an increased incidence of male infants being born with cryptorchidism, a condition in which the testicles do not descend into the scrotum but remain undescended inside the abdomen.

Another study found that there has indeed been a huge decrease over the last fifty years in the quality of human semen. (A recent study measuring sperm quality in New York City contradicted these findings; however, the problem remains that there is great variability in such studies.) There has also been a huge increase in the incidence of testicular and prostate cancers. In Britain, testicular cancer incidence has tripled over the last fifty years. It is now the most common cancer in young men under age 30. In Denmark, there has been a 400 percent increase in testicular cancer. As for prostate cancer, its incidence has doubled over the last decade. These male reproductive problems have been linked to environmental estrogens, too.

The scientific literature is slowly becoming saturated with finings linking one organic chemical after another to reproductive cancers and "endocrine disruption" in both wildlifeandhumans. It appears that organic chemicals are transforming into environ-mental estrogens. Organic chemicals are in the air we breathe from numerous air pollutants, in the food preservatives used in numerous canned and packaged goods, and in the pesticides used on fresh produce. These chemicals then contaminate the water and soil, which contaminate the entire human food chain.

It has been suggested that environmental estrogens are "feminizing" the planet. It is suggested that women are being overloaded with estrogen, which may be associated with the rise of estrogen-dependent cancers, such as ovarian and breast cancer, as well as estrogen-related conditions, such as endometriosis (an estrogenic condition where pieces of the uterine lining grow outside the uterus and can block the fallopian tubes) and fibroids. Estrogen pollutants are also thought to accumulate in fatty tissues (meaning they are stored in fat). Since women generally carry more body fat than men, women may be accumulating more of these toxins. Some studies have already found that women with breast cancer tend to have higher concentrations of the organochlorines DDT, DDE, or PCBs in their fat tissue. In fact, elevated levels of DDE in the blood have been directly linked to a fourfold increase of breast cancer in the United States. We already know that dioxins, which are also organochlorines, are associated with endometriosis. (However, dioxin has antiestrogen effects that can cause a decrease in breast cancer.)

Some suggest that the picture is equally dismal for men, many of whom are not only becoming slowly sterilized by this phenomenon but are also developing reproductive cancers. Several prominent scientists have gone on record to say that the estrogen problem is the environmental priority of the twenty-first century.

On the flip side, many doctors point out that in the Western world, there has also been a huge increase in the "fatness" of the population. This also increases the level of estrogen produced by our bodies.

What About the Children?

Cancer rates among North American children under the age of 15 have increased by roughly 25 percent within the last 25 years; the highest rates of childhood cancer are seen in children under age 5. Cancer is considered to be the second major cause of death in children after accidents. The lifestyle of toddlers has not changed much over the past half century. Young children do not smoke, drink alcohol, or hold stressful jobs. Children do, however, receive a greater dose of whatever chemicals are in the air, food, and water because, pound for pound, they breathe, eat, and drink more than adults do.

Source: Sandra Steingraber. Living Downstream. *Addison-Wesley (1997):39.*

What Can Our Governments Do About This?

Ideally, our governments ought to act on many of the following recommendations, which are based on previous proposals by state/provincial, national, and international bodies. Some of these recommendations address the problem of persistent toxic chemicals in general; others deal separately with specific known or suspected carcinogens. In some cases, dealing with groups of substances at a time (such as those at work in incinerators, landfills, or vehicle emissions) is a better strategy. Controlling the level of toxic chemicals in our air, water, soil, and food supply can only have a positive effect on the control of specific known or suspected carcinogens. It is not only our governments that are spending time trying to ensure that the world is safe from dangerous chemicals. In May 2004, the city of Louisville, Kentucky, hosted a meeting of a whole network of people who had the common goal of protecting human health and ridding the world of unnecessary toxic chemicals. Meeting in this city had particular resonance, since, as they note on their Web site "Louisville, Kentucky, USA, is home to the area known as 'Rubbertown,' which has eleven industrial facilities releasing millions of pounds per year of toxic air emissions—one-third of all reported toxic releases in Kentucky." Together, this group produced the Louisville Charter for Safer Chemicals (www.louisvillecharter.org), with the goal of becoming the basis for policy making at all levels of government, and that ultimately, perhaps, a reformed national chemical policy could evolve from the ideas generated here. This is truly impressive grassroots action at the local level.

Changing the Standards of Proof

One of the most important changes governments can make to protect public health is to change their standards of proof. Right now, governments like conclusive proof that a chemical or substance is toxic or harmful before they ban it. This isn't realistic. Instead, governments ought to withhold approval of chemicals for use until there is conclusive proof that they are safe. Erring on the side of caution is the best policy. As noted on the Greenpeace Web site (www.greenpeace.org), "Scientific uncertainty is not a reason to proceed with a potentially harmful activity until such time as the extent of harm becomes clearer. On the contrary, it should be a reason to be cautious because what we do not know is more than what we know." In other words, chemicals should be "suspected carcinogens" until they are proven to be noncarcinogenic. This is especially important for new substances. This policy won't help reduce the amount of persistent toxic substances already in use, but it will, at least, prevent more from being added to the environment. That said, we can certainly ban the import of persistent toxic substances. (There are no "air borders," of course, but we can ban certain produce known to be sprayed with certain pesticides, and so forth.)

Sunsetting

Sunsetting is a step-by-step process that aims to restrict, phase out, and one day ban the production, generation, use, transport, storage, discharge, and disposal of a persistent toxic substance. Sunsetting involves two things:

1. It targets the chemical and the manufacturing and production processes associated with that chemical.

2. It looks at ways of eliminating the substance within realistic parameters.

Reducing the Health Risks

Instead of ignoring the health risks associated with environmental contaminants the population is facing, governments should face them and deal with them. Some ways to deal with them include:

- Making the pollution prevention agencies work with industrial policy authorities so that the technology of business and the technology of research share some common ground

- Adopting the rigorous standards for controlling environmental carcinogens developed by Organization for Economic Cooperation and Development (OECD) member nations
- Making a list of what is toxic, suspected to be toxic, and definitely not toxic so everyone knows. The Ontario Ministry of Environment and Energy's "Candidate Substances for Bans, Phase-Outs or Reductions" is a good example of this.
- Banning organochlorines. Knowing what we do about organochlorines, how can we still allow them into our atmosphere? Many contend that there are chlorine compounds that can be used safely. Chlorine has a preventive side, too. It is commonly used for water purification, needle sterilization, and chlorinated pharmaceutical production. But perhaps those benefits can be found using a different process or noncarcinogenic chemical. Perhaps we need to deal with organochlorines as a class of toxic chemicals, and sunset them accordingly. In establishing a timetable for sunsetting, them, we may want to think about first banning those organochlorines that are themselves carcinogenic, or those that have been known to introduce carcinogens into the environment.

Banning All Carcinogenic Pesticides

There are noncarcinogenic pesticides that we can use these days. The use of suspected carcinogenic pesticides has contaminated both our environment and our food chain. A number of pesticides that are known animal and suspected human carcinogens are actually registered as legal for use. Another more achievable goal would be to restrict use so we know how much we're using and where it is used. Much work has been done in the area of banning pesticides, even down to the level of individual homes. In the agricultural sphere, the U.S.-based group called the Pesticide Action Network (PAN) at www.panna.org, which has been lobbying for alternatives to pesticides worldwide for twenty-five years, helps to bridge public discourse and grassroots activites around the issue of pesticide bans.

Contamination occurs differently than you might think. It's not that the food we eat contains detectable residues of harmful organochlorines because it's been sprayed with pesticides; rather that these substances have started to accumulate in our surface water, groundwater, sediment, soil, and air. It is this concentration within the food chain of bioaccumulative substances that poses the greatest threat to human health.

It's estimated that billions of gallons of toxic pesticides have been released into an unsuspecting environment. Since these chemicals are resistant to breaking down, as mentioned above, they're spread around the world through the air and water, exposing us to these poisons in our food, groundwater, surface water, and air. According to a Greenpeace report on chlorine and human health, no industrial organochlorines are known to be nontoxic.

The consumption of certain popular food products containing the residues of twenty-eight different pesticides has been blamed on some twenty thousand excess cancer deaths in the United States each year. This is a controversial estimate, however, and many believe it should be used only in relation to preventive dietary measures (if you eat your fruits and veggies, their protective factor will overwhelm the cancer-causing hazards of pesticide residues in foods).

To further address cancer risks associated with exposure to pesticides, experts recommend:

- Developing and applying alternative, nonchemical pest-control methods, such as those used by organic growers
- Sunsetting the following chemicals, which meet IARC/USEPA (U.S. Environmental Protection Agency) criteria for known or suspected carcinogens, still registered for use across North America:

  » Group 2A (probable human carcinogens): ethylene oxide (insecticide, fungicide), formaldehyde (antimicrobial), creosote (wood preservative).
  » Group 2B (possible human carcinogens): amitrole (herbicide), atrazine (herbicide), dichlorvos (insecticide), hexachlorocyclo-hexanes (lindane–gamma-HCH, insecticide, acaricide), pentachlorophenol (wood preservative), sodium ortho-phenylphenate (antimicrobial).

Reducing Radiation Risks

In order to control the cancer risks associated with hazardous levels of radiation, and to start identifying where unrecognized hazards from exposure might occur, experts recommend:

- Developing an inventory of sources of radioactive nuclides in the United States and Canada
- Investigating how radioactive substances travel through the food chain
- Imposing "chemical control rules" for suspected radioactive contaminants, which would result in more stringent standards
- Studying radioactive emissions from energy production plants
- Investigating ways of phasing out these materials wherever an increased cancer risk is found

Reducing Car Exhaust

Car exhaust is making us sick. Cancer is just one of many health risks linked to motor vehicle emissions today.

Ground-level ozone is created when volatile organic compounds meet nitrogen oxides (found in emissions from burning fossil fuels), and has been associated with lung diseases and other respiratory problems. Worst of all, car exhaust leads to "earth sickness" because it is the ground-level ozone from motor vehicle emissions that causes both global warming and acid rain. Put the two together, and the damage to the ecosystem may be irreparable. To reduce car exhaust from our lives, here are some steps many governments are already taking:

- Decrease emissions from all sources. That includes from cars, trucks, and motorcycles as well as two-stroke engines (such as lawn mowers, chainsaws, minibikes, motorboats, and some mopeds) that emit benzene and PAHs.
- Test vehicles regularly for hazardous levels of emissions. (California is already seeing huge improvements in its air quality through this measure.)
- Start gasoline vapor recovery programs at all fuel transfer facilities and gas stations to reduce unwanted benzene emissions. (This is in place in several areas across North America; California was one of the first to implement it and is seeing the positive results.)
- Support research on the development of alternative, environmentally friendly fuels (such as hydrogen) that reduce the overall impact on the environment
- Encourage people to change the way they get to work (for example,

walking, cycling, or using public transit)

- Subsidize less-polluting forms of travel. This could mean anything from decreased public transit fares to newer, more accessible bicycle lanes. The point is to discourage urban sprawl and subsidize public transit.
- Engage in judicious urban planning so that more people can afford to live close to where they work and shop (big box stores are the wrong way to go)

Hybrid Cars

Hybrid cars have become more and more accessible and affordable in the last few yearswhich also save gas, and therefore popular for economic reasons, too. For more information, visit: www.fueleconomy.gov.

Creating New Jobs Through Alternative Safe Substances

Governments can get industry on board by creating incentives for developing alternatives to the toxic substances now in use. Many European countries, for example, are developing feasible, cost-effective alternatives to some of the toxic substances currently used and produced in North America. Since the whole world is concerned, new alternatives could mean big bucks for the manufacturers or creators of those alternatives. North American governments ought to look at environmentally friendly initiatives as "job creation" rather than "job destruction" initiatives. That said, by eliminating many of these persistent toxic substances, jobs will be affected. Therefore, our governments can:

- Develop transition plans to aid those who will be adversely affected by the elimination of the use and production of these substances
- Create a taxation scheme whereby taxes are increased in small increments to provide economic incentives for the reduction of toxic emissions during the phase-out period. In Britain, for example, excise duties have been adjusted so that the price of leaded gas has risen increasingly, relative to the price of unleaded. Partly as a result, lead

155

emissions from the exhausts of British cars fell by 70 percent in the decade up to 1990. When Sweden introduced a charge of $6,000 per ton on nitrous oxide emissions from power stations in 1992, average emissions fell 35 percent within two years. A Swedish tax on the sulfur content of diesel fuel resulted within eighteen months to a tenfold increase in the share of "clean" diesel in total diesel consumption.

- Develop a fund from those tax revenues to help in the transition to a less toxic industrial society. The funds could be used to explore and demonstrate economically viable alternatives and, again, to aid those workers who have lost their jobs as a result of the transition.

Supporting Public Education Initiatives

The public has a right to know what is going on. Educational programs (including public reports on health and the environment) would be better off addressing the spectrum of issues stemming from environmental health concerns, rather than focusing specifically on cancer. To increase public awareness of environmental health issues, governments can:

- Continue to develop environmental health sciences programs at the grade-school level, teaching students how environmental science works, and how relationships between health and the environment work. The Washington State Department of Ecology, for example, (www.ecy.wa.gov) has an entire Web page devoted to assisting teachers with creating a classroom curriculum in environmental sciences. They list teacher workshops, reference and research materials, as well as a listing of grant opportunities funded by public agencies and nonprofit groups. Industry can help fund special programs in this area, too.
- Encourage university-age students to go into the environmental sciences so they can help solve tomorrow what we can't solve today
- Support nongovernmental groups and organizations in their efforts to educate the public and to develop community action plans
- Support community action plans that encourage prevention
- Support intersectoral (meaning, multiple industries coming together) activities on environment and health

HOW CAN WE HELP OURSELVES?

The first thing we can do to help ourselves is to send the message to our governments and industries that we can't afford to wait for the science. Because we don't yet know the extent to which environmental contaminants contribute to cancer, public health and health promotion experts agree that the only prudent approach to safeguarding the health of the general public is to be precautionary and wait until research makes us sure. In other words, we should presume the guilt of a potentially toxic substance before we judge it to be innocent. Don't release it into the atmosphere until it's proven safe. This is a "science will follow" versus "no danger yet" approach. For now, we ought to demand policies that protect the public from any known or suspected human and animal carcinogens, as no dose of a carcinogen can be considered a safe dose.

Finding Out the Facts

Consumers have a right to know the following:

- Known and suspected environmental carcinogens
- The cancers associated with each environmental carcinogen
- What science can prove and what it can't prove (as mentioned earlier, it's difficult to absolutely prove certain links because of the way we are trained to research, and because sometimes there are just too many variables involved)
- The other health risks (e.g., reproductive disorders) posed by environmental carcinogens
- Strategies already in place for reducing or, where possible, eliminating exposure to environmental carcinogens

Limiting Your Exposure

The best place to start the environmental cleanup is in your kitchen. Your weekly groceries probably contain residues from pesticides and other organochlorines (on store-bought fruits and vegetables), hormones in meat products, as well as a number of "extras" you may not have bargained for, which were fed to your meat when it was still alive. These include feed additives, antibiotics, and tranquilizers. Meanwhile, anything packaged will most likely contain dyes and flavors from a variety of chemical concoctions.

Airborne contaminants, waste, and spills affect the water and soil, which affect everything we ingest. When one species becomes unable to reproduce, we could lose not just that species but all those that depend on it, thus disrupting the food chain. Cleaning up the food chain is all part of creating a healthy, contaminant-free diet for ourselves. So make the following grocery list before your next shopping trip:

- You can find out what your produce has eaten, and whether it was injected with anything by contacting the U.S. National Food Safety Database at www.foodsafety.gov. or the Canadian Food Inspection Agency at www.cfia-acia.agr.ca
- You can find out what waters your fish has swum in by contacting the previously mentioned organizations.
- You can find out what your produce was sprayed with by contacting the previously mentioned organizations.
- You can find "safe food" that is organically grown or raised through a number of natural produce supermarkets or get in touch with the Organic Trade Association (serving both Canada and the United States) at www.ota.com. You can also support your local farmers' market. To find one closest to you in the United States, check the Web site www.localharvest.org. You can find out more about your supermarket's buying habits when it comes to produce by contacting your supermarket's head office.

The Natural Resources Defense Council (www.nrdc.org) contains a wealth of information about food facts your supermarket may not tell you about. For example, you'll learn about the environmental costs of food transport over eating locally. In 2005, the import of fruits, nuts, and vegetables into California by airplane released more than 70,000 tons of CO_2, which is equivalent to more than 12,000 cars on the road." These are startling statistics that most of us do not contemplate during our excursions to the grocery store.

Read Any Good Labels Lately?

Are you worried about the plastic that lines certain canned goods? Demand labeling that identifies the organic chemicals used to make that plastic. Worried about the plastics used in various cosmetics, detergents, and spermicides? What exactly is plastic wrap made out of anyway? You have a right to know. What was this spinach sprayed with? You have a right to a label that reads: "This produce sprayed with endosulfan." Many chemical ingredients that make up plastic products are kept from the consumer because they're considered trade secrets. This is unacceptable. Many websites such as www.foodnavigator.com should become as routine as reading the paper, which pulls together hundreds of food news for the average consumer.

In Your Own Backyard

While you might have a beautiful flower garden that may be the envy of all your neighbors, if you're using pesticides, you're part of the problem, not the solution, as they said in the 1960s. The Organic Trade Association (www.ota.com) has lots of literature available on organic insecticides and fungicides for lawns and gardens, as well as companion planting tips for the backyard (such as planting garlic beside roses).

Learning More About Bioengineered Food

Genetically altered produce and animals (where genes are manipulated for different growth results) are seen as one way to get around pesticides and diseases while improving food delivery. Scientists are concerned that by dicing and splicing various genes, ecological Frankensteins could be introduced into the environment, creating opportunities for exotic organisms and diseases to wreak havoc on our health. For example, in an effort to create strawberries that can grow in frost conditions, bioengineers unwittingly created a weed that can also grow in frost, which can interfere with other plants. Cloning is widespread in agriculture and farming. There is the potential for bioengineered foods and genetic engineering to create very good things for the future. Scientists can clone extra organs or perhaps find better treatments for cancer or completely reinvent farming and do away with pesticides. But we ought to support this research in controlled laboratories. Right now, consumers are often unwitting and unwilling research participants in an ongoing experiment as we are buying altered fruits and vegetables that are not labeled as such. U.S. consumers were alarmed in 2007, for example, to hear that cloned meat may be sold to supermarkets without proper labeling. The FDA has been following this issue, and an archive of statements and testimony on this topic can be viewed here: www.fda.gov/newsevents/testimony/ucm112927.htm.

The danger is in allowing these new breeds of plants or animals to breed or pollinate with their "original" species, spoiling the gene pools ever after. To find out whether your produce was genetically engineered, check the Food and Nutrition page at the USDA (www.usda.gov) or for Canada, go to www.agr.gc.ca.

Food Made in China

A new issue of concern in the last few years has been the safety of food, medicine, and other products from foreign countries. China, in particular, has been the focus of great concern, especially when in early 2007 reports were coming in about toxic pet food ingredients making their way into the United States from China, causing the deaths of numbers of dogs and cats. A *Washington Post* story on May 20, 2007, sounded the alarm with the title: "Tainted Chinese Imports Common." The story goes on to say:

> Dried apples preserved with a cancer-causing chemical. Frozen catfish laden with banned antibiotics. Scallops and sardines coated with putrefying bacteria. Mushrooms laced with illegal pesticides. These were among the 107 food imports from China that the Food and Drug Administration detained at U.S. ports just last month, agency documents reveal, along with more than 1,000 shipments of tainted Chinese dietary supplements, toxic Chinese cosmetics, and counterfeit Chinese medicines.

The uncertainty these days over the safety of foreign food imports makes the safety of domestically grown products all the more crucial.

Learn More

The International Agency for Research on Cancer (IARC) provides up-to-date data on suspected or known environmental carcinogens. For a complete list of agents and mixtures that are possibly, probably and known-to-be carcinogenic to humans visit: http://monographs.iarc.fr.

GREAT LAKES, BIG MESS

The Great Lakes Basin is home to some 40 million people, which is 30 percent of Canada's population and 10 percent of the U.S. population, and is the largest body of freshwater on earth. If you're living in any of the eight Great Lakes U.S. states (Minnesota, Wisconsin, Michigan, Illinois, Indiana, Ohio, New York, and Pennsylvania), or in Ontario, your health is at risk due to the presence of several hundred contaminants in the Great Lakes Basin, a dozen of which have been identified as really serious, such as PCBs and dioxins. The contaminant levels in the breast milk of women living in these regions show that for suckling infants, the daily intake of PCBs and dioxins (or dioxinlike contaminants) may exceed established guidelines for human exposure. But the alternative to breastfeeding —formula feeding—has even more serious health consequences for babies. More babies will die from digestive problems associated with formula than from the contaminants they're exposed to through breastfeeding, so health promotion experts still recommend breastfeeding to women living in these regions.

Another health paradox looms in the Great Lakes Basin: eating fish from the Great Lakes is a major source of carcinogens in local residents because these toxins bioaccumulate in the fish. But, for so many of us, heart-smart diets depend on consuming fish oils from fatty fish—the very fish that swim in the Great Lakes. We need these good fats to protect us from heart disease, so we must weigh the risks of contamination against the risk of heart disease. There are no easy answers other than trying to clean up the mess. What are the health consequences of Great Lakes toxins? In terms of cancer, we are looking at higher incidences of breast, testicular, and prostate cancers due to the estrogenic toxins (i.e., toxins that break down into an estrogenic mimic) that are rampant in the Great Lakes waters. Other cancers, such as bladder, thyroid, and colon, are also elevated in these regions. There are higher risks of infertility in this population. Women are more likely to develop endometriosis and fibroids, which thrive on estrogen. In one study surveying 575 couples trying to conceive who regularly ate fish from heavily polluted Lake

Ontario, they were 25 percent less likely to conceive each month. New York State has been advising women of childbearing age to avoid Lake Ontario fish for some time.

Lake Ontario is known for its high concentrations of PCBs and other compounds, which can have hormonelike effects that disrupt a woman's fertility. As the International Joint Commission (IJC) 12th Biennial Report on Great Lakes Water Quality (www.ijc.org/php/publications/html/12br/english/report/index.html) notes "Pathogens enter the Great Lakes ecosystem from surface runoff and erosion from farm manure stockpiles, sludge applications, overflows or spills from holding pens or ponds, and storage lagoons, all of which can leach into soil and ground water." It is no small wonder that there are toxic consequences to this runoff into our Great Lakes. Researchers from the State University of New York at Buffalo published the findings of this study in the July 2000 issue of *Epidemiology*. Meanwhile, Great Lakes baby boys are more likely to be born with undescended testicles, and then, as adults, could even be infertile due to low sperm counts. Fetuses exposed to these toxins are at greater risk for developmental disabilities. We also have too much harmful bacteria floating around, which come from the sewage pumped into these waters over the years. These are public health hazards, too. For example, no one has been allowed to swim in most parts of Lake Ontario for years.

A BRIEF HISTORY OF GREAT LAKES WATER QUALITY

Just in case you're not a geography whiz, the Great Lakes comprise Lake Ontario (the source of the St. Lawrence River), Lake Erie, Lake Huron, Lake Michigan, and Lake Superior. These waters and the lands that drain into these waters form what is known as the Great Lakes Basin, and when discussing environmental concerns, the term *Great Lakes Basin ecosystem* is used. This is a huge territory that consists of area in eight U.S. states and the province of Ontario, plus Quebec, which is connected to the basin through the St. Lawrence River. A number of large industrial cities lie along the Great Lakes, which are connected to the Mississippi River and the Gulf of Mexico by the Illinois River waterway.

In the 1970s, the term *water pollution* was often used to describe many of the issues in this chapter. That term has been replaced with the term *water quality*. So what's the definition of good water quality? Well, good water quality in this case means that the chemical, physical, and biological integrity of the waters of the Great Lakes Basin ecosystem is intact and not damaged. In other words, we have poor water quality in the Great Lakes Basin ecosystem because the chemical, physical, and biological integrity of the waters has been damaged, with detrimental effects on the surrounding wildlife and human life.

The Great Lakes have always raised concerns between the United States and Canada. The Boundary Waters Treaty of 1909 was created to prevent and resolve water resource disputes along the boundary between the two countries. Even as early 1909, there was a commitment not to pollute the boundary waters "to the injury of health or property on the other site."

Unfortunately, both countries broke this commitment as industry and cities were built around the Great Lakes Basin. The peak water-polluting years were between 1950 and 1975. Many of the substances polluting the Great Lakes come from the air in the form of industrial and municipal discharges that come down in the rain; sources are widespread in North America and beyond. The lakes recirculate previously deposited pollutants from cities and industries, as well. A concerted effort was made to clean up the water, and between 1972 and 1994, pollutants directly deposited into the Great Lakes were cut in half. Unfortunately, pollutants released into the air almost doubled. In Ontario, roughly 99 percent of the pollutants damaging the Great Lakes are coming from air emissions. The Canadian National Pollutant Release Inventory and the U.S. Toxics Release Inventory report similar findings, and estimate that between 73 and 85 percent of pollutants in the Great Lakes Basin are in the air (calculations vary depending on whether one is calculating on a per day basis). Factor in emissions from electric power utilities and municipal incinerators, and the air pollutants increase substantially.

1972: The Year of Watergate . . . and Water Quality
The first Great Lakes Water Quality Agreement was signed between Canada and the United States in 1972 (ironically to coincide with Watergate!). This was essentially a pollution control agreement between President Richard Nixon and Prime Minister Pierre Trudeau. The good news is that today the Great Lakes Basin ecosystem is actually cleaner than it was two decades ago. And the U.S.-Canada "clean-up team-up" proves that governments can do something about these messes.

The bad news is that the Great Lakes were so problematic in the 1970s that, while cleaner, they're still not clean enough. We're still dealing with lingering problems, and feeling the health effects today. For example, we have not yet eliminated the persistent toxic substances that both governments agreed to eliminate back in 1978. Both countries can also jeopardize the good work that has been done through cutbacks in environmental legislation, regulation, and funding for monitoring, enforcement, and research.

Less than Zero

In 1995, U.S. president Bill Clinton and Canadian prime minister Jean Chrétien announced an agreement to develop a binational strategy for the virtual elimination of persistent toxic substances in the Great Lakes Basin. The two countries came up with a target list of chemicals, which could have promising results. The chemicals on the list were targeted for *virtual elimination*, meaning the release of persistent toxic chemicals due to human activity must be stopped. This hasn't happened yet. *Zero discharge* means no discharge of persistent toxic substances resulting from human activity. This hasn't happened yet, either. In the past, these goals have been distorted to mean "less" activity or discharge by private industry. Anything less than zero is still a problem.

In the early 1990s, Lake Superior was designated a "demonstration area" for virtual elimination and zero discharge, meaning no persistent toxic substance would be permitted. Ontario, Michigan, Minnesota, and Wisconsin (where Superior flows) committed to the Binational Program to Restore and Protect Lake Superior. So far, there have been great plans for this Great Lake, with not much action.

Great Lakes Water Quality Agreement of 1978

To meet their commitments to the water quality agreement of 1978, both the United States and Canada invested in sewage treatment facilities, storm water runoff management, and controls for discharges coming from industry. The countries also began banning phosphorus and certain pesticides.

However, there are a number of activities in both countries that are reversing hard-won progress, such as:

- Relaxed pollution control policies and relaxed enforcement, including reporting and compliance requirements
- Lack of funding and expertise for much-needed research, monitoring, and enforcement. For example, the U.S. Clean Water Act is undergoing statutory review, whereby "self-audits" by various jurisdictions are being favored over federal supervision.
- Reviews, revisions, and legislative riders that weaken or even eliminate existing environmental laws. A case in point is the U.S. Toxic Substances Control Act (TSCA) that was originally designed to prevent additional toxic contaminants from entering the environment and to address the risks posed by existing chemicals. Approximately 72,000 chemicals are on TSCA chemicals list, but revised regulations call for a control of only nine new chemicals in twenty years, limiting control to only polychlorinated biphenyls (PCBs). Yet, there are far more toxic substances to contend with than PCBs. Similar limitations exist in Canada through the Canadian Environmental Protection Act (CEPA). This act is currently applied to a relatively small number of listed substances, using the chemical-by-chemical approach instead of the class-of-chemicals approach.

We don't know enough about our Great Lakes fish, but instead of solving the problem by establishing the research resources to study the fish and learn about their toxicity levels, governments are cutting resources. For example, funds have been cut from the Great Lakes fish tissue specimen bank. This is where researchers get their fish samples so that they can monitor and assess the impact of persistent toxic chemicals on the fish. Samples are kept over the years so that comparisons can be made between, say, a second millennium fish and a late 1980s fish. We need to keep this kind of research going if we want to keep eating salmon and trout. In the United States, the Agency for Toxic Substances and Disease Registry (ATSDR) may also lose funding. This is a crucial registry that studies people who consume Great Lakes fish for epidemiological studies (the study of diseases by groups of people).

In other cases, enforcement responsibilities are being left to other levels of government without the resources for adequate enforcement.

Worst Areas

The Great Lakes Basin is divided into *areas of concern* and *areas of quality*. The areas of concern include Green Bay–Fox River; Duluth, Minnesota; Ashtabula, Ohio; Toronto Bay; and Hamilton Harbor. *The IJC Report*, (p. 47) notes that: "Environmental problems in the Lake Erie ecosystem function as early warning signals for the other Great Lakes. As the shallowest of the lakes, Lake Erie has the shortest water retention time (less than three years), but it also has the largest watershed relative to its size, the highest human population density, the most farm land, and the largest number of major cities. These factors converge to make Erie the Great Lake where ecological disruption often shows up first." Altogether, in the Great Lakes Basin, there are forty-three areas of concern (AOCs). Areas are ranked by how many species are declining or living in degraded conditions, whether the nutrients in the area are in good or bad shape, and how many contaminants are affecting wildlife and human health. To date, many AOCs are due for upgrades, and haven't had them yet. As a step forward, the Great Lakes Legacy Act (http://epa.gov/greatlakes/sediment/legacy/index.html) was signed into law in 2002 to tackle the problem areas in the Great Lakes that have been identified. Thirty-one of the forty-three AOCs have been identified as being located on the U.S. side of the Great Lakes. The Legacy Act provides the necessary funds in order that steps can be taken to clean up contamination specifically in the AOCs in the United States.

A CATALOG OF PROBLEMS

Anyone living in the Great Lakes Basin depends on its ecosystem for drinking water and fresh fish. As explained earlier, persistent toxic substances are largely organochlorines, a class of toxins that include pesticides and PCBs, dioxins, furans, and similar substances, which break down into an estrogen-like substance that is being linked to a host of estrogenic cancers, as well as to poor sperm counts and hermaphroditic traits in many fish and wildlife species.

In the 1980s, many Great Lakes fisheries were closed down because dangerous substances such as mercury and PCBs were found in lake trout and salmon. In the mid-1990s, a retrospective risk assessment suggested that dioxin in Lake Ontario may have caused complete reproductive failure in native lake trout populations in the early 1940s. Today, lake trout is usually produced through fish farming, known as "artificial stocking," which hasn't proved to be the best alternative (trout prefer their natural habitat). There are some exciting improvements to report, however, as far as how fish are doing in the Great Lakes. An Environment Canada press release from 2005 reported that since governments began implementing fishing quotas, in an attempt to reduce pollution and to control invasive species, "some native fish are making a comeback." Furthermore, the press release reports that pike are again swimming in Toronto Harbor, and that "an artificial reef is being built off Detroit's shoreline to facilitate the return of the sturgeon . . . and lake trout, after nearly being wiped out in much of the Great Lakes, are now able to survive in Lake Superior and parts of Lake Huron."

As you may recall from the previous chapter, food contamination has far-reaching social consequences, too. Contamination of perch, the dietary staple on the Akwesasne Reserve, led to widespread chronic health problems among the residents there.

These toxins are not limited to the Great Lakes, however. Although the Great Lakes are heavily contaminated, humans have managed to pollute just about every source of water on the planet. For example, pesticides were found in a lake on Isle Royale at concentrations higher than those in the surrounding waters of Lake Superior. They've also been found bodies of water in Florida, the Netherlands, and the Arctic. It is a global problem that is magnified in the Great Lakes Basin. What goes on in the Great Lakes Basin is an example of what goes on in other waters.

Who's Most at Risk for Great Lakes Health Problems?

Some people are more at risk for Great Lakes health problems than others:

- *People who consume a large amount of Great Lakes fish.* Those at greatest risk for health problems are those who consume fish they have caught themselves (people who fish for livelihood or sport). Aside from sport fishermen, people who depend on catching their own fish to survive are often poor, with no access to "safe fish" that have passed inspection by fisheries (which actually may not mean much). You can view the government of Canada's "Guide to Eating Ontario Sport Fish" (www.ene.gov.on.ca/envision/guide/index.htm). A similar document from New York State entitled "Health Advice on Eating Sportfish and Game," can be obtained at www.health.ny.gov/environmental/outdoors/fish/health_advisories/docs/advisory_booklet.pdf

- *Fetuses.* When exposed to toxic chemicals in utero, fetuses can be born with developmental disabilities as well as reproductive health problems, such as undescended testicles. One study involved human infants in upper New York State whose mothers ate Lake Ontario salmon prior to pregnancy. The findings (reported in 1995) suggest that behavioral abnormalities are more prevalent in the babies born to this group of women. And, in fact, the same behavioral abnormalities were found fifteen years ago in babies born to a group of mothers who ate Lake Michigan fish.

- *Breastfed children.* Again, breast milk can pass on levels of toxins that exceed guidelines for human health.

- *People who drink untreated water in the Great Lakes Basin.* Members of this group are exposing themselves to a host of bacterial, viral, and protozoan contamination, which can lead to gastrointestinal illnesses.

- *People who swim in these waters.* They are at risk of contamination through swallowing water or skin exposure—bathing, boating, or other water sports on the Great Lakes can increase exposure to toxins.

Sources of Priority Contaminants and Routes of Exposure

Contaminant	Sources	Routes of Human Exposure
Polychlorinated biphenyls (PCBs)	Used in electrical trans-formers and capacitors, and in hydraulic equipment; also as lubricants and heat-transfer fluids. Released to environment primarily from equipment in use and by waste site leakage.	Consumption of contaminated foods, particularly fish, meat, and dairy products.
Polychlorinated dibenzo-*p*-dioxins (PCDDs) (especially 2,3,7,8- TCDD) an dipolychlorinated dibenzofurans (PCDFs)	Formed as impurities during the synthesis of various chlorinated compounds (e.g., certain pesticides and herbicides); released through pulp and paper bleaching and solid waste incineration; found in exhaust from vehicles using fossil fuels; and can also result from the combustion of any chlorinated organic material.	Consumption of contaminated foods, particularly fish, meat, and dairy products.
Dichlorodiphenyl trichloroethane (DDT) and its degradation products e.g., DDE	An insecticide now banned in Canada and the U.S. Sources are leakage from waste sites and atmospheric transport and deposition.	Consumption of contaminated foods, especially fish and dairy products.
Mirex	A fire retardant and contact insecticide once used in Canada and the U.S. but now banned. Extremely persistent; may reach the GLB via surface run-off from contaminated soils or by leaching from hazardous waste sites.	Consumption of contaminated foods.
Toxaphene	An insecticide used on cotton fields. Its use is restricted in Canada and the U.S. Sources include contaminated soils, hazardous waste sites, and air transport.	Consumption of contaminated foods.

Contaminant	Sources	Routes of Human Exposure
Aldrin and Dieldrin (i.e., chlorinated cyclodienes. Other examples are chlordane and its metabolites, heptachlor and heptachlor epoxide)	Aldrin and dieldrin are insecticides used for control of soil insects and mosquitos. Dieldrin is also produced from the metabolic oxidation of aldrin. Their use is restricted.	Consumption of contaminated foods especially fish.
Hexachlorobenzene (HCB)	A fungicide no longer used in Canada or the U.S.; also generated as a by-product of fuel combustion and the production of some pesticides.	Consumption of contaminated foods especially fish.
Hexachlorocyclo-hexanes (HCHs) e.g., lindane	An insecticide, lindane is one of the 8 HCH isomers. HCH is the key isomer found in human tissue, accumulating in body fat. No longer produced in the U.S., but still in use as an import. Registered for use in Alberta.	Consumption of contaminated foods. Can be transported by water and air.
Microbial contaminants e.g., bacteria, viruses, protozoa	Found in poorly treated sewage discharge, agricultural run-off and urban run-off; also storm water run-off, animal feces.	Consumption of contaminated drinking water or recreational water; absorption through breaks in skin.
Radionuclides	Natural radiation comes primarily from radioactive elements in the earth's crust, with additional minor contributions from cosmic rays and cosomogenic radionuclides. Anthropogenic sources include nuclear weapons test fallout and emissions from nuclear fuel cycle operations.	Inhalation of contaminated air and consumption of contaminated food and water (internal dosing), and exposure by direct irradiation (external dosing).

Contaminant	Sources	Routes of Human Exposure
Methylmercury (MeHg)	Biosynthesis as result of atmospheric deposition of elemental mercury from natural oceanic output (30–40% of annual Hg emissions to atmosphere); released from inundated vegetation. Inorganic Hg occurs naturally in soils and as a by-product of chlor-alkali, paint, and electrical equipment production processes. MeHg bioconcentrates in fish.	Consumption of contaminated fish and marine products.
Cadmium	Waste dumps and waste incinerators, fertilizers, sewage, sludge, solid wastes, cadmium mining/refining operations, soil, plant-life, atmospheric deposition.	Consumption of contaminated foods, esp. organ meats (liver, kidney), seafood (shellfish, crustaceans), and cereals (e.g., wild rice); tobacco use, consumption of drinking water (minor).
Lead	Combustion of leaded gasoline, metal smelters, automotive batteries, contaminated soil and dust, lead-based paints, drinking water in contact with lead-soldered pipes, atmospheric deposition.	In the absence of a point source of contamination, consumption of contaminated foods and drinking water; inhalation of contaminated air.
Ground-level Ozone	Formed from the interaction of nitrogen oxides and hydrocarbons in the atmosphere in presence of sunlight. Can be transported long distances.	Inhalation of contaminated air.

Contaminant	Sources	Routes of Human Exposure
Acid Aerosols	Formed when pollutants such as sulphur dioxide and oxides of nitrogen are transformed in the atmosphere in the presence of sunlight; may be transported long distances from original source in the form of rain, snow, vapor, fine particles and gases; can be both air and water pollutants.	Inhalation of contaminated air.
Airborne particles	Very small pieces of solid or liquid matter that vary in size, chemical composition and source. Can be course of fine. Fine particles arise mainly from man-made sources such as combustion of fuels, and include sulphates and nitrates as well as metals. Coarse particles consist largely of naturally occurring substances, particularly soil.	Inhalation of contaminated air.
Polycyclic Aromatic Hydrocarbons (PAHs) e.g., benzo[a]pyrene	Incomplete combustion of fossil fuels, organic matter, and solid waste; combustion activities associated with industry (e.g., coke production, metal smelting, oil refining). Non-commercial sources include wood-burning fireplaces, cigarette smoke, vehicle exhaust; and smoked, grilled, fried, or barbecued meat and fish.	Inhalation of contaminated air and consumption of certain foods.

174

Contaminant	Sources	Routes of Human Exposure
Volatile organic compounds (VOCs) e.g., trihalomethanes, benzene, trichloroethylene	Formed from natural or industrial sources by the interaction of chlorine with organic materials; also found in dry-cleaning solvents; both an airborne and drinking water contaminant.	Inhalation of contaminated air from exposure to chlorinated tap water during showering, bathing or to dry-cleaning solvents, and consumption of drinking water.

Source: Great Lakes Health Effects Program 1993

Routes of Contamination

How do contaminants from the Great Lakes get into our bodies? Here are all the ways it can happen:

- Food and fish. While Michigan fish advisories may ban one kind of toxic fish, Ontario fish advisories may allow the sale of that same fish. So the first order of business is for all eight Great Lakes states and Ontario to agree on which fish to ban, and which fish to sell.
- Drinking water
- Milk
- Our skin (through dermal exposure)
- Inhalation

Tests done on bodily secretions and excretions (urine, feces, saliva, breast milk, or sweat) have confirmed the presence of toxins from all of these sources; additional tests on hair samples have also added verification. When you mix airborne contaminants with the "lake effect" winds, it contributes to ozone depletion, smog, and acid rain, which gets directly into our crops and other vegetation— and then hits the food chain.

Radioactive Substances

Where there is lots of water, there are lots of nuclear power stations! And that means there is concern about the potential for nuclear accidents and core water being dumped into the lakes. There is also concern about the production, use, and storage of radioactive materials and nuclear wastes, as well as what to do about *decommissioned* nuclear power stations. Radioactive materials get discharged into the Great Lakes and affect our health, which can lead to a number of cancers. But the problem is that there is no comprehensive inventory of how many radioactive substances are released around the Great Lakes Basin.

Other Great Lakes Problems

Cancer increases notwithstanding, here are some other serious problems in the Great Lakes Basin.

Natural Habitat

We need to save the Great Lakes natural habitat, and we need to have healthy plant life to support its aquatic life and wetlands creatures. At least fourteen species of fish and fish-eating wildlife in the region suffer from serious reproductive problems. The U.S. Fish and Wildlife Service has listed twenty-two endangered and/or threatened species in the Great Lakes that are affected by poor water quality.

According to Environment Canada reports, the entire shorelines of Lake Ontario, Lake Erie, and southern Lake Huron are destroying numerous species due to pesticide use by agriculture. Even with various programs in place, both the Canadian and U.S. governments are starting to have more relaxed standards for habitat protection.

Biocontamination

Biocontamination occurs when nonnative wildlife or plant species are introduced into a new area, destroying or interfering with native wildlife or plant species. Over the last hundred years, roughly

140 nonnative or exotic species have been introduced into the Great Lakes region, which include the infamous purple loosestrife (a colorful weed that wreaks havoc with other plant life), as well as the zebra mussel. Zebra mussels caused the extinction of native clams in Lake Erie in less than a decade. As a result, smelt and yellow and white perch are now endangered species; when species begin to disappear, it's a sign that the health of the environment is in question. The IJC report from 2004 notes on page 15, that despite encouraging initiatives from various organizations, the flow of new invasive species to the Great Lakes has, in fact, not been stopped. The report estimates that "more than 170 non-indigenous fish, invertebrates, plants, algae, protozoa and parasites, and predict that one new non-indigenous species will be discovered in the lakes about every eight months." These invaders can prove to be ecologically destructive to the fragile system.

Nonnative species come from ships and unwittingly stow away as water from one region gets shipped into other waters (called ballast water). This is how young flounder got into Thunder Bay and Lake Erie. By pumping out ballast water before the ship's old water is introduced into new water, we can control this growing problem. And again, climate changes are starting to make the Great Lakes Basin attractive to more exotic species.

Lake Ontario Biomagnification of PCBs
As PCBs work their way up the food chain, their concentrations in animal tissue can be magnified up to 25 million times. Microscopic organisms pick up persistent chemicals from sediments (a continuing source of contamination) and water, and are consumed in large numbers by filter-feeding tiny animals called zooplankton. Larger species like mysids then consume zooplankton, fish eat the mysids, and so on up the food chain to the herring gull.

WHAT TO REQUEST FROM THE GREAT LAKES BUSINESS COMMUNITY

Many of the suggestions made in chapters 7 and 8 for getting businesses—primarily industry—on board with cancer prevention programs are relevant here, too, as we're dealing with the same issues: trying to eliminate airborne toxins and persistent toxic substances, while stopping the release of any new substance until it's been proven safe. In addition, it's important to contact local businesses and insist they be aware of the environmental practices of anyone they are partnering with outside of Canada and/or the United States. When we import contaminated products from other countries, we contaminate our own country. There are also some specific requests we must make of Great Lakes businesses and industries:

- *Find alternatives to polyvinyl chloride (PVC), which is mostly manufactured and used in the Great Lakes Basin.* Currently, the industry states that its production and use is harmless and even environmentally beneficial, that PVC is a stable product and its manufacture does not cause pollution. But experts are concerned about PVC's eventual disposal and destruction through incineration or the open environment.
- *Encourage small businesses to join cleanup programs.* Small businesses are often missed by government programs and trade associations. The dry-cleaning industry, for example, uses solvents that pose a hazard to the environment, as well as to customers and employees. Other small industries include the printing and graphic arts industry, automotive products, auto body repair, the manufacture and installation of floor coverings, photography labs, and machine components. Pay attention to what kinds of illnesses are prevalent in different businesses. If statistics aren't kept, find out why not. Alternative processes are imperative, and can be developed if enough consumers, like you and me, complain. Small businesses can be supported through government incentive programs or grants to retrofit (upgrade) to environmentally sound processes.

- *Lobby for the use of "green" products.* Businesses large and small, plus their customers (that's us), must support one another in purchasing environmentally friendly products.
- *Request public environmental accountability.* All businesses should produce separate environmental annual reports that provide public accountability regarding how they are contributing to virtual elimination and zero discharge.
- *Develop measures to ensure compliance.* The IJC Report states: "regulating agencies should be able to evaluate ballast water discharges for the presence of aquatic alien invasive species. Ideally, this technology could be used to establish financial liability for damages arising from biological pollution." This measure could ultimately make the shipping companies much more responsible in the Great Lakes waters.

Fishing for Funding

One of the most natural places to petition for funding Great Lakes Basin cleanup programs of any sort are the fish-related industries. A letter requesting funding or volunteers from any of the following businesses, with a reminder of how they can capitalize on the good PR a cleanup program will generate, is an excellent start. These businesses can also join in partnership with the government to help fund educational initiatives.

- Frozen-fish food manufacturers
- Fish/seafood restaurants
- Fishing-supplies companies, retailers, or manufacturers
- Hotel and tourism industries that specialize in boating or fishing sports
- Boating manufacturers
- Water-sports manufacturers

WHAT TO RECOMMEND TO YOUR GREAT LAKES GOVERNMENT

If you are one of the residents affected by the Great Lakes issues, it's up to you and me to lobby our local governments for the following:

- *Funding for continued enforcement of the Great Lakes Water Quality Agreement and other pro-environmental policies in the Great Lakes Basin.* We need to reverse the recent trend of cutting funding rather than providing it. To obtain a copy of the Great Lakes Water Quality Agreement, visit www.great-lakes.net. Lakewide Management Plans (LAMPS) are local programs that focus on specific areas in the Great Lakes Basin that can help to police certain areas and enforce aspects of the Great Lakes Water Quality Agreement. Experts have been recommending LAMPS for years, but so far there is a lack of funding and action to get them started. The IJC Report mentions a 2004 Executive Order signed by President Bush that created a U.S. Great Lakes Interagency Task Force intended to improve interagency regional coordination. This action was, in turn, welcomed by Canada's Minister of the Environment.
- *Funding and programs to restore areas of concern*
- *Funding for health risk education programs for Great Lakes residents, particularly for citizens living in areas of concern.* We need to be informed of the health risks we are facing so that we can make healthier lifestyle choices, and perhaps go for regular screenings for at-risk cancers.
- *Education for healthcare providers (especially in areas of concern) so that they can help to validate complaints of ill health, and be more prudent in referring people for regular screening for certain cancers that are more prevalent in those areas.* This entails support from universities, environmental health chairs in professional schools of health sciences, research and teaching hospitals, and related businesses, such as the pharmaceutical industry. We need more healthcare practitioners who are informed, up-to-date, and knowledgeable about environmental medicine. Physician groups such as the American College of Occupational and Environmental Medicine (www.acoem.org) "represents more than 5,000 physicians and other healthcare

professionals specializing in occupational and environmental medicine." Round tables and workshops need to be coordinated along with support from the Canadian Great Lakes Health Effects Program and the U.S. Agency for Toxic Substances and Disease Registry (ATSDR).

- *The establishment of Environmental Health as a credible medical specialty that can attract young doctors to train in it.* Perhaps more schools like New York University School of Medicine will open up programs such as its Department of Environmental Medicine, which was founded in 1947. (See www.med.nyu.edu/environmental.) It is one of the country's oldest and most important centers for research into the health effects of environmental pollution.

- *Fishing education programs to warn people who sport-fish of the dangers of contaminants and the routes of fish contamination.* These programs can also include labels that identify risky fish so that we can choose other foods.

- *A list of known pollutants coming into the Great Lakes Basin from both Canada and the United States for constituents and consumers*

- *More research programs to examine toxins in the Great Lakes Basin and how they affect our health.* Areas that desperately need to be researched are human health effects, water conservation, and cleanup technologies in areas of concern. Again, universities and private business can help to fund research.

- *A reduction in incineration.* Again, a lot of water pollutants start in the air, particularly through municipal, industrial, and medical/hospital incinerators. Right now, waste management programs allow and even encourage incineration. Although newly upgraded incinerators are okayed by governments, the results are not okay. We need alternatives to incineration if we want to reduce pollutants in the Great Lakes Basin.

- *A decrease in mercury.* Mercury mainly comes from thermal power stations. We need to find ways of reducing mercury emissions, which have serious health consequences.

Cleaning up the Great Lakes is a long process, and a long time coming, but we cannot deny the increased cancer risks and other health problems in the Great Lakes Basin. In the 1980s, we all learned the three R's (Reduce, Reuse, and Recycle) to help reduce the amount of garbage being poured into landfill sites. In the new millennium, we need to learn two P's: Precaution (proving a chemical is safe before use instead of proving it guilty later) and Phase Out by Class (pulling categories of chemicals from the shelves, not just single chemicals).

In the 1980s, eleven critical pollutants were identified by the Great Lakes Water Quality Board:

- PCBs
- DDT and its metabolites
- Dieldrin
- Toxaphene
- Mirex
- Dioxin
- Furans
- Benzopyrene
- Hexachlorobenzene
- Lead
- Mercury

Health Canada also identified radionuclides, airborne contaminants, and microorganisms as being problematic. Many of these substances are still in the environment. Some are still being produced and are waiting for their final sunset. And in the meantime, there are several hundred contaminants in the Great Lakes Basin that freely persist.

Note: This chapter is based on the recommendations of the Twelfth Biennial Report *on Great Lakes Water Quality, Under the Great Lakes Water Quality Agreement of 1978 to the Governments of the United States and Canada and the State and Provincial Governments of the Great Lakes Basin, released by the International Joint Commission, available at: www.ijc.org/php/publications/html/12br/english/ report. It also includes information from a unique 1998 report entitled* A State of Knowledge Report on the Effects of Human Health in the Great Lakes Basin, *published by Health Canada in cooperation with the Great Lakes Health Effects Program, Environmental Health Effects Division of Health Canada.)*

BIBLIOGRAPHY

Accelerated Reduction/Elimination Toxics. *ARET Candidate Substances List.* Hull, Quebec: ARET, 1994.

Action on Smoking and Health. "Pipe and cigar smoking: The report of an expert group appointed by Action on Smoking and Health." *Practitioner* 210 (1973): 645–648.

Advisory Committee on Environmental Standards. *A Standard for Tritium: A Recommendation to the Minister of Environment and Energy.* Toronto: ACES Report 94-01, 1994.

Agriculture Canada. *Ontario Farm Groundwater Quality Survey.* Ottawa, 1993.

Alavanja, M., R. C. Brownson, J. L. Lubin, et al. "Residential radon exposure and lung cancer among nonsmoking women." *Journal of the National Cancer Institute* 86 (1994): 1829–1837.

Albandar J. M., C. F. Streckfus, M. R. Adesanya, and D. M. Winn. "Cigar, pipe, and cigarette smoking as risk factors for periodontal disease and tooth loss." *Journal of Periodontology* 71 (2000): 1874–1881.

American Institute for Cancer Research. *Food, Nutrition, Physical Activity, and the Prevention of Cancer.* 2007.

Ayanian, John Z., Betsy A. Kohler, Toshi Abe, and Arnold M. Epstein. "The relation between health insurance coverage and clinical outcomes among women with breast cancer." *New England Journal of Medicine* 329 (1993): 326–331.

Bailar, John C., III, and Heather Gornick. "Cancer Undefeated." *New England Journal of Medicine* 336 (1997): 1569–1574.

Barker, D. J. P., et al. "Poor housing in childhood and high rates of stomach cancer in England and Wales." *British Journal of Cancer* 61 (1990): 675–678.

Bartlett, J. G. "Epidemiology and clinical aspects of antibiotic-associated colitis." Proceedings of the 2nd International Symposium on Anaerobes, June 22, 1985, Tokyo.

Bates, D., and R. Sitzo. "Air pollution and hospital admissions in Southern Ontario: the acid summer haze effect." *Environmental Research* 4 (1987): 203–22.

Belpomme, D., P. Irigaray, L. Hardell, et al. "The multitude and diversity of environmental carcinogens." *Environ Research* 105 (2007): 414–429.

Benowitz, N. L. "Pharmacologic aspects of cigarette smoking and nicotine addiction." *New England Journal of Medicine* 310 (1988): 1318–1330.

Beral, V., and N. Robinson. "The relationship of malignant melanoma, basal and squamous skin cancers to indoor and outdoor work." *British Journal of Cancer* 44 (1981): 886–892.

Bergkvist, L. H. O., I. Adami, R. Persson, R. Hoover, and C. Schairer. "The risk of breast cancer after estrogen and estrogen-progestin replacement." *New England Journal of Medicine* 321 (1989): 293–297.

Black, D., et al. *The Black Report (Report of the Working Group on Inequalities in Health)*. London: DHSS, 1980.

Bryden, W. L. "Mycotoxins in the food chain: human health implications." *Asia Pacific Journal of Clinical Nutrition* 16 (2007): 95–101.

Bondy, M., and C. Mastromarino. "Ethical issues of genetic testing and their implications in epidemiologic studies." *Annals of Epidemiology* 7 (1997): 363–366.

Bove, C. M., et al. "Presymptomatic and predisposition genetic testing: ethical and social considerations." *Seminars in Oncology Nursing* (1997): 135–140.

Britt, Beverley, Dr. "Pesticides and Alternatives." Excerpted from the Canadian Organic Growers Toronto Chapter's Spring Conference: 1–4.

Cancer 2000 Task Force. *Inequalities in Cancer Control in Canada*. Ottawa: Cancer 2000 Task Force Panel on Cancer and the Disadvantaged, 1992.

Caplan, L. S. "Disparities in breast cancer screening: is it ethical?" *Public Health Review* 25 (1997): 31–41.

Carlson, C. "A comprehensive school-based substance abuse program with cooperative community involvement." *Journal of Primary Prevention* 10 (1990): 289–302.

Carmichael, J. A., and P. D. Maskens. "Cervical dysplasia and human papillomavirus." *American Journal of Obstetrics and Gynecology* 160 (1989): 916–918.

Caygill, C. P., et al. "Occupational and socioeconomic factors associated with peptic ulcer and with cancers following consequent gastric surgery." *Ann Occ Hyg* 34 (1990): 19–27.

Centers for Disease Control. "Cancer and steroid hormone study. Combination oral contraceptives use and the risk of ovarian cancer." *JAMA* 249 (1983): 1596–1599.

Centers for Disease Control. "Cancer and steroid hormone study. Combination oral contraceptives use and the risk of ovarian cancer." *JAMA* 257 (1987): 796–800.

Centre for Health Promotion, Department of Public Health Sciences, University of Toronto. "Proceedings of a Conference on the Effect of Hormonal Disrupters on the Health and Development of Children," June 25, 1999.

Chief Medical Officer of Health. *Progress Against Cancer*. Toronto: Ministry of Health, 1994.

Colborn, Theo, J. P. Myers, and Dianne Dumanoski, *Our Stolen Future*. New York: Dutton, 1996.

Colborne, T., and C. Clement. *Chemically-Induced Alterations in Sexual Functioning and Development: The Wildlife-Human Connection*. Princeton, NJ: Princeton Scientific Publishing Co., 1992.

Colorectal Cancer Screening. Final Report of the Ontario Expert Panel, April 1999.

Colorectal Dis. 2005 May; 7(3): 04–13.

Committee on Diet and Health. *Diet and Health: Implications for reducing chronic disease risk*. Washington, D.C., National Academy Press, 1989.

Cooke, K. R., D. C. G. Skegg, and J. Fraser. "Socio-economic status, indoor and outdoor work and malignant melanoma." *International Journal of Cancer* 37 (1984): 57–62.

Council on Scientific Affairs. "Cancer risk of pesticides in agricultural workers." *JAMA* 260 (1988): 959–966.

Daling, J. R., K. E. Malone, L. F. Voigt, et al. "Risk of breast cancer among young women: relationship to induced abortion. *Journal of the National Cancer Institute* 86 (1994): 1584–1592.

Darbre, P. D. "Underarm cosmetics and breast cancer." *Journal of Applied Toxicology* 23 (2003): 89–95.

Davies, D. L., A. Blair, and D. G. Hoel. "Agricultural exposures and cancer trends in developed countries." *Environmental Health Perspectives* 100 (1992): 39–44.

Davies, D. L., et al. "Medical hypothesis: xenoestrogens as preventable causes of breast cancer." *Environmental Health Perspectives* 101 (1993): 372–377.

Davies, K. "Concentrations and dietary intake of selected organochlorines, including PCBs, PCDDs and PCDFs in fresh food composites grown in Ontario, Canada." Chemosphere 17 (1988): 263–276.

Davies, K. *Human exposure routes to selected persistent toxic chemicals in the Great Lakes Basin.* Toronto: City of Toronto Department of Public Health, 1986.

De Sanjose, S., et al. "Association between personal use of hair dyes and lymphoid neoplasms in Europe." *American Journal of Epidemiology* 164 (2006): 47–55.

Delmas, C., C. Platat, B. Schweitzer, et al. "Association between television in bedroom and adiposity throughout adolescence." *Obesity* 15 (2007): 2495–2503.

Dewailly, E., S. Dodin, R. Verault, et al. "High organochlorine body burden in women with estrogen receptor-positive breast cancer." *Journal of the National Cancer Institute* 86 (1994): 232–234.

Dickens, Bernard M., Nancy Pei, and Kathryn M. Taylor. "Legal and Ethical Issues in Genetic Testing and Counseling for Susceptibility to Breast, Ovarian, and Colon Cancer." *Canadian Medical Association Journal* 154 (1996): 813–818.

Doll, R., and R. Peto. "The causes of cancer: quantitative estimates of avoidable risks of cancer in the United States today." *Journal of the National Cancer Institute* 66 (1981): 1191–1308.

Draelos, Z. D. "Self-tanning lotions: are they a healthy way to achieve a tan?" *American Journal of Clinical Dermatology* 3 (2002): 317–318.

Edwards, G. *Alcohol Policy and the Public Good.* Oxford: Oxford University Press, 1994.

Ekbom, A., et al. "Evidence of prenatal influences on breast cancer." *Lancet* 340 (1992): 1015–1018.

Elwood, J.M., et al. "Sunburn, suntan and the risk of cutaneous malignant melanoma: the Western Canada Melanoma study." *British Journal of Cancer* 35 (1985): 427.

Environment Canada. *A Primer on Ozone Depletion.* Ottawa (1993).

Environmental and Occupational Working Groups of the Toronto Cancer Prevention Coalition. *Preventing Cancer From Environmental and Occupational Factors: A Strategy for the City of Toronto.* March 7, 2000.

Environmental Health Program of the Environmental Defense Fund. *Executive Report* (1997).

Epstein, S. S. "Evaluation of the national cancer program and proposed reforms." *International Journal of Health Services* 23 (1993): 15–44.

Epstein, S. S. *The Politics of Cancer.* New York: Anchor Books, 1979.

Epstein, Samuel S., and David Steinmean with Suzanne LeVert, *The Breast Cancer Prevention Program: The First Complete Survey of the Causes of Breast Cancer and the Steps You Can Take to Reduce Your Risks.* New York: Macmillan, 1998.

Farley, T. A., and J. T. Flannery. "Late-stage diagnosis of breast cancer in women of lower socioeconomic status: public health implications." 79 (1989): 1508–1512.

Ferlin, A., D. Zuccarello, A. Garolla, et al. "Hormonal and genetic control of testicular descent." *Reproductive Biomedicine Online* 15 (2007): 659–665.

Feychting, M., and U. Forssen. "Electromagnetic fields and female breast cancer." *Cancer Causes Control* 17 (2006): 553–558.

Filby, A. L., T. Neuparth, K. L. Thorpe et al., "Health impacts of estrogens in the environment, considering complex mixture effects." *Environmental Health Perspective* 115 (2007): 1704–1710.

Flack, F., et al. "Pesticides and PCB residues in human breast lipids and their relation to breast cancer." *Archives Environmental Health* 47 (1992):143–146.

Frank, R., et al. "Organochlorine residues in adipose tissues, blood and milk from Ontario residents, 1976-1985." *Canadian Journal of Public Health* 79: 150–158.

Fulkerson, J. A., and S. A. French. "Cigarette smoking for weight loss or control among adolescents: gender and racial/ethnic differences." *Journal of Adolescent Health* 32 (2003): 306–313.

Funch, D. P. "Socioeconomic status and survival for breast and cervical cancer." *Women and Health* 11 (1986): 37–54.

Funch, D. P. "A Report on cancer survival in the economically disadvantaged." Prepared for the American Cancer Society Subcommittee on Health Care of Economically Disadvantaged Cancer Patients, 1985.

Ghadirian, P., J. P. Thouez, and A. Simard. "La geographie du cancer de l'oesophage." *Social Science and Medicine* 27 (1988): 971–985.

Gofman, John W. *Preventing Breast Cancer: The Story of a Major, Proven, Preventable Cause of This Disease*. San Francisco: CNR Book Division, Committee for Nuclear Responsibility, 1995.

Gorham, B. D., C. F. Garland, and F. C. Garland. "Acid haze, air pollution and breast and cancer colon cancer mortality in twenty Canadian cities." *Canadian Journal of Public Health* 80 (1989): 96–100.

Gottileb, M. S., et al. "Lung cancer in Louisiana: death certificate analysis." *Journal of the National Cancer Institute* 63 (1979):1131–1137.

Griffith, J. L., et al. "Cancer mortality in U.S. counties with hazardous waste sites and environmental pollution." *Archives Environmental Health* 44 (1989): 69–74.

Halpern, M. T., B. H. W. Gillespie, and K. E. Warner. "Patterns of absolute risk of lung cancer mortality in former smokers." *Journal of the National Cancer Institute* 85 (1993): 457–464.

Hancock, T. "Sustaining Health: Achieving Health for All in a Secure Environment." Paper presented at the Conference on Health-Environment-Economy, York University, Toronto, April 1989.

Harvey, P. W., and Philippa Darbre. "Endocrine Disrupters and Human Health: Could Oestrogenic Chemicals in Body Care Cosmetics Adversely Affect Breast Cancer Incidence in Women? A Review of Evidence and Call for Further Research." *Journal of Applied Toxicology* 24 (2004): 167–176.

Hatch, M. C., et al. "Cancer rates after the Three Mile Island nuclear accident and proximity of residence to the plant." *American Journal of Public Health* 81 (1991): 719–724.

Hayes, H. M., et al. "Case control study of canine malignant lymphoma: positive association with dog owner's use 2,4-dichlorophenoxyacetic acid herbicides." *Journal of the National Cancer Institute* 83 (1991): 1226–1231.

Henley, S. J., M. J.Thun, A. Chao, and E. E. Calle. "Association between exclusive pipe smoking and mortality from cancer and other diseases." *Journal of the National Cancer Institute* 96 (2004): 853–861.

Henriksen, T., et al. "Ultraviolet-radiation and skin cancer: effect of an ozone layer depletion." *Photochem Photobiol* 51 (1990): 579–582.

Hill, D., V. White, and N. Gray. "Australian patterns of tobacco smoking in 1989." *Medical Journal of Australia* 154 (1991): 797–801.

Holick, M. F. "Sunlight and vitamin D for bone health and prevention of autoimmune diseases, cancers, and cardiovascular disease." *American Journal of Clinical Nutrition* 80 (2004): 1678S–1688S.

Holmes, M. D., and W. C. Willett. "Does diet affect breast cancer risk?" *Breast Cancer Research* 6 (2004): 170–178.

Holtzman, N. A. "Medical and ethical issues in genetic screening—an academic view." *Environmental Health Perspective* 104 (1996): 987–990.

Horstman, D., W. McDonnell, et al. "Changes in pulmonary function and airway reactivity due to prolonged exposure to typical ambient ozone levels." In T. Schneider et al., eds., *Atmospheric Ozone Research and its Policy Implications. Amsterdam*: Elsevier, 1989.

Howe, G. R., J. D. Burch, A. B. Miller, et al. "Tobacco use, occupation, coffee, various nutrients, and bladder cancer." *Journal of the National Cancer Institute* 64 (1980): 701–713.

Hunter, J. E., and T. H. Applewhite. "Reassessment of Trans Fatty Acid Availability in the U.S. Diet." *American Journal of Clinical Nutrition* 54 (1991): 363–369.

IARC. IARC Monographs on the Evaluation of Carcinogenic Risks of Chemicals to Humans. Vol. 44. *Alcohol Drinking*. Lyon: International Agency for Research on Cancer, 1988.

IARC . IARC Monographs on the Evaluation of Carcinogenic Risks of Chemicals to Humans. Vol. 59. *Hepatitis Viruses*. Lyon: International Agency for Research on Cancer, 1994.

IARC Study Group on Cancer Risk among Nuclear Industry Workers. "Direct estimates of cancer mortality due to low doses of ionizing radiation: an international study." Lancet 34 (1994): 1039–1043.

IARC. IARC Monographs on the Evaluation of Carcinogenic Risks of Chemicals to Humans. Vol. 38. Tobacco Smoke. Lyon: International Agency for Research on Cancer, 1986.

IARC. IARC Monographs on the Evaluation of Carcinogenic Risks of Chemicals to Humans. Vol. 42. *Silica and Some Silicates*. Lyon: International Agency for Research on Cancer, 1987.

IARC. IARC Monographs on the Evaluation of Carcinogenic Risks of Chemicals to Humans. Vol. 60. *Some Industrial Chemicals*. Lyon: International Agency for Research on Cancer, 1994.

IARC. IARC Monographs on the Evaluation of Carcinogenic Risks of Chemicals to Humans. Vol. 61. *Schistosomes, Liver Flukes and Helicobacter Pylori*. Lyon: International Agency for Research on Cancer, 1994.

Industrial Disease Standards Panel. *Report to the Workers' Compensation Board on Lung Cancer in the Hardrock Mining Industry*. IDSP Report No. 12, Toronto, 1994.

Infante, P. F., and G. K. Puhl. "Living in a chemical world: actions and reactions to industrial carcinogens." *Teratogenesis Carcinog*. Mutagen 8 (1988): 225–249.

International Food Information Council. Antibiotics in Animals: *An Interview with Stephen Sundlof*, D.V.M., Ph.D. Washington, D.C., 1997.

International Joint Commission, Canada and the United States. *Twelfth Biennial Report on Great Lakes Water Quality*. September 2004.

International Joint Commisssion, Canada and the United States. *Thirteenth Biennial Report on Great Lakes Water Quality*. December 2006.

International Joint Commission. *Sixth Biennial Report on Great Lakes Water Quality*. Windsor, Ontario: International Joint Commission, 1992.

Internationa Joint Commission. *Eighth Biennial Report On Great Lakes Water Quality, Under the Great Lakes Water Quality Agreement of 1978 to the Governments of the United States and Canada and the State and Provincial Governments of the Great Lakes Basin*. Windsor, Ontario: International Joint Commission, 1996.

Irigaray, P., J. A. Newby, R. Clapp, et al. "Lifestyle-related factors and environmental agents causing cancer: an overview." *Biomedicine & Pharmacotheraphy* 61 (2007): 640–658.

Journal of Clinical Gastroenterolology 41, no.8 (September 2007): 731–746.

Jones, R. R. "Ozone depletion and cancer risk." *Lancet* 2 (1987): 443–446.

Journal of Clinical Oncology 21, no. 12 (June 2003): 2397–2406.

Kaldor, J. M., N. E. Day, and S. Shiboski. "Epidemiological studies of anti-cancer drug carcinogenicity." In Schmael, D., and J.M. Kaldor, eds., Carcinogenicity of alkylating cytostatic drugs. IARC scientific publications no. 78. Lyon: Intl Agency for Research on Cancer, 1986.

Keiding, L. M. "General preventive measures against carcinogenic exposure in the external environment." *Pharmacology and Toxicology* 72 (1993):s136–s138.

Kendall, P. "City of Toronto Dept. Pub. Health presentation to the Standing Committee on the Environment and Sustainable Development of the House of Commons." Toronto, Ontario (1994).

Khlat, M. "Mortality from melanoma in migrants to Australia: variation by age of arrival and duration of stay." *American Journal of Epidemiology* 135 (1992): 103.

Kjaer, S. K., P. Poll, H. Jensen, et al. "Abnormal Papanicolau smear. A population-based study of risk factors in Greenlandic and Danish women." *Acta Obstet Gynecol Scand* 69 (1990): 79–86.

Koutsky, L. A., D. A. Galloway, and K. K. Holmes. "Epidemiology of genital human papillomavirus infection." *Epidemiological Reviews* 10 (1988): 122–163.

Kreiger, N., M. S. Wolff, R. A. Hiatt, et al. "Breast cancer and serum organochlorines: a prospective study among white, black and Asian women." *Journal of the National Cancer Institute* 86 (1994): 589–599.

Krewski, D., B. W. Glickman, R. W. Habash, et al. *Journal of Toxicology and Environmental Health* 19 (2007): 287–318.

Kuczmarski, R. J., K. M. Flegal, S. M. Campbell, and C. L. Johnson. "Increasing Prevalence of Overweight Among U.S. Adults: The National Health and Nutrition Examination Surveys, 1960 to 1991. *Journal of the American Medical Association* 272 (1994): 205–211.

Kusiak, R.A., J. Springer, et al. "Carcinoma of the lung in Ontario gold miners: possible aetiological factors." *British Journal of Industrial Medicine* 48 (1991): 808–817.

Labonte, R., and K. Davies. "Stop the carcinogens." *Policy Options* 7 (1986): 33–57.

Lancet 371, no. 9612 (February 16, 2008): 569–578

Landrigan, P. L. "Environmental disease: a preventable catastrophe." *American Journal of Public Health* 82 (1992): 941–943.

Le Foll, B., and T. P. George. "Treatment of tobacco dependence: integrating recent progress into practice." *CMAJ* 177 (2007):1373–1380.

Leon, D. A. *The Social Distribution of Cancer, Longitudinal Study* 1971–1975. London: HMSO Series LS No. 3, 1988.

Letourneau, E. G., D. Krewski, N. W. Choi, et al. "Case-control study of residential radon and lung cancer in Winnipeg, Manitoba, Canada." *American Journal of Epidemiology* 140 (1994): 310–322.

Levi, F., et al. "Socioeconomic groups and cancer risk: a death at the Swiss Canton at Vaud." *International Journal of Epidimiology* 17 (1988): 711–717.

Lindheim, R., and S. L. Syme. "Environments, people and health." *Annual Review of Public Health* 4 (1983): 335–359.

Loh, M. M., J. I. Levy, J. D. Spengler, et al. "Ranking cancer risks of organic hazardous air pollutants in the United States." *Environmental Health Perspective* 115 (2007): 1160–1168.

Longnecker, M. P. "Alcoholic beverage consumption in relation to risk of breast cancer: meta-analysis and review." *Cancer Causes and Control* 5 (1994): 73–82.

Magano, J. J. "Cancer mortality near Oak Ridge, Tennessee." *International Journal of Health Services* 24 (1994): 521–533.

Maltoni, C., and I. J. Selikoff. "Living in a chemical world: occupational and environmental significance of industrial carcinogens." *Annals New York Academy of Science* 534 (1988): 1–1045.

Marrett, L. D., et al. "The use of host factors to identify people at high risk for cutaneous malignant melanoma." *Canadian Medical Association Journal* 147 (1992): 445–453.

Martin, K. A., and M. W. Freeman. "Postmenopausal hormone-replacement therapy." *New England Journal of Medicine* 328 (1993): 1115–1117.

Mayer, J. A., D. J. Slymen, E. J. Clapp, et al. "Promoting sun safety among U.S. Postal Service letter carriers: impact of a 2-year intervention." *American Journal of Public Health* 97 (2007): 559–565.

McGinnis, J. M., and W. H. Foege. "Actual causes of death in the United States." *JAMA* 270 (1993): 2207–2212.

McTiernan, A. "Mechanisms linking physical activity with cancer." *National Review of Cancer* (2008).

McWhorter, W. P., et al. "Contribution of socioeconomic status to black/white differences in cancer incidence." *Cancer* 63 (1989): 982–987.

Meen, Elizabeth, "Ex-Bell employees uncover high levels of cancer at Hamilton office." *The Expositor*, May 7, 1998.

Mendoza, J. A., F. J. Zimmerman, and D. A. Christakis. "Television viewing, computer use, obesity, and adiposity in U.S. preschool children." *International Journal of Behavioral Nutrition* 4 (2007): 44.

Michaud, D. S., E. A. Platz, and E. Giovannucci. "Gonorrhea and male bladder cancer in a prospective study." *British Journal of Cancer* 96 (2007): 169–171.

Michels, K. B., A. P. Mohllajee, E. Roset-Bahmanyar, et. al. "Diet and breast cancer: a review of the prospective observational studies." *Cancer* 109 (2007): 2712–2749.

Millar, J. "Sex differentials in mortality by income level in urban Canada." *Canadian Journal of Public Health* 74 (1983): 329–334.

Miller, A. B. "An overview of hormone-associated cancers." *Cancer Res* 38 (1978): 3985–3990.

Miller, A. B. "Asbestos fiber dust and gastro-intestinal malignancies. Review of literature with regard to a cause/effect relationship." *J Charon Dis* 31 (1978): 23–33.

Miller, A. B. "Planning cancer control strategies." *Chronic Diseases in Canada* 13 (1992): s1–s39.

Miller, A. B. "Risk/benefit considerations of antiestrogen/estrogen therapy in healthy postmenopausal women." *Preventive Medicine* 20 (1991): 79–85.

Miller, A. B., F. Berrino, M. Hill, et al. "Diet in the aetiology of cancer: a review." *European Journal of Cancer* 30 (1994): 207–220.

Miller, A. B., G. Anderson, J. Brisson, et al. "Report of a national workshop on screening for cancer of the cervix." *Canadian Medical Association Journal* 145 (1991): 1301–1325.

Mills, P. K., R. Yang, and D. Riordan. "Lymphohematopoietic cancers in the United Farm Workers of America (UFW), 1988–2001." *Cancer Causes Control* 16 (2005): 823–830.

Minister of Health, Minister of Public Works and Government Services Canada. *State of Knowledge Report on Environmental Contaminants and Human Health in the Great Lakes Basin.* Catalogue Number H46-2/97– 214E, 1997.

Morris, R. D., et al. "Chlorination, chlorination by-products and cancer: a meta-analysis." *American Journal of Public Health* 82 (1992): 955–963.

Muir, C. S., and A. J. Sasco. "Prospects for cancer control in the 1990s." *Annual Review of Public Health* 11 (1990): 143–163.

Mustard, J. F., E. Farber, A. B. Miller, D. McCalla, and J. E. Till. *Report of the Special Advisory Committee on Carcinogens. Fourth Annual Report of the Advisory Council on Occup Hlth and Occup Safety,* 1981–1982. (1982).

National Academy of Sciences. *Potential Risk of Lung Cancer from Diesel Engine Emissions.* Washington, D.C.: National Academy Press, 1981.

National Academy of Sciences. *Regulating Pesticides in Food: The Delaney Paradox.* Washington D.C.: National Academy Press, 1987.

National Cancer Institute of Canada. "Canadian cancer statistics, 1995." Toronto, 1995.

National Cancer Institute. *Bioassay of Chlordane for Possible Carcinogenicity.* Bethesda, MD: Carcinogenesis Technical Report Series 8, 1977.

National Coalition Against the Misuse of Pesticides (U.S.). Testimony of NCAMP before the Senate Subcommittee on Toxic Substances, Environmental Oversight, Research and Development, Committee on Environment and Public Works, 1981.

National Council of Welfare. *Health, Health Care and Medicare: A Report by the National Council of Welfare.* Ottawa: Ministry of Supply and Services, 1990.

National Institute for Occupational Safety and Health Carcinogenic Effects of Exposure to Diesel Exhaust. Bethesda, MD: NIOSH Current Intelligence Bulletin 50, 1988.

Nightingale, T. E., and J. Gruber. "Helicobacter and human cancer." *Journal of the National Cancer Institute* 86 (1994): 1505–1509.

Nsubuga, J. "Organochlorine residues and breast cancer risks in women." *PHERO* (1993): 170–172.

Onstot, J. R., R. Ayling, and J. Stanley. *Characterization of HRRC/CCMS Unidentified Peaks from the Analysis of Human Adipose Tissue.* Washington, D.C.: U.S. EPA 560 / 6-87-002a, 1987.

Ontario Ministry of Agriculture and Food, and Ministry of the Environment. *Polychlorinated Dibenzo-P-Dioxins and Polychlorinated Dibenzofurans and Other Organochlorine Contaminants in Food.* Toronto: Queen's Printer for Ontario, 1988.

Ontario Ministry of Environment and Energy. *Candidate Substances for Bans, Phase-Outs or Reductions.* Toronto: Queen's Printer for Ontario, 1993.

O'Reilly, K. M., A. M. Mclaughlin, W. S. Beckett, and P. J Sime. "Asbestos-related lung disease." *American Family Physician* 75 (2007): 683–688.

Ozonoff, D. "Taking the Handle of the Chlorine Pump." Presentation made at Public Health Forum, Boston University School of Public Health, October 5, 1993.

Pearce, N. E., and J. K. Howard. "Occupation, social class and male cancer mortality in New Zealand 1974-78." *Int J Epid* 15 (1986): 456–462.

Preston, D. S., and R. S. Stern. "Nonmelanoma Cancers of the skin." *New England Journal of Medicine* 327 (1992): 1649–1661.

Pukkala, E., and L. Teppo. "Socioeconomic Status and Education as Risk Determinants of Gastrointestinal Cancer." *Preventive Medicine* 15 (1986): 127–138.

Qureshi, A. M., and H. E. Robertson. "Polychlorinated byphenyls (PCB) in breast milk from Regina nursing mothers." *Canadian Journal of Public Health* 78 (1987): 389–392.

Rabkin, C. S., and F. Yellin. "Cancer incidence in a population with a high prevalence of infection with human immunodeficiency virus type 1." *Journal of the National Cancer Institute* 86 (1994): 1711–1716.

Rall, D. "Laboratory animal toxicity and carcinogenesis testing: underlying concepts, advances and constraints." *Annals New York Academy of Science* 534 (1988): 78–83.

Raloff, J. "That feminine touch." *Science News* 145 (1994): 56–59.

Rimpela, A. H., and E. I. Pukkala. "Cancers of affluence: positive social class gradient and rising incidence trend in some cancer forms." *Soc Sci Med* 24 (1987): 601–606.

Risch, H. A, L. D. Marrett, and G. R. Howe. "Parity, contraception, infertility, and the risk of ovarian cancer." *American Journal of Epidemiology* 140 (1994): 585–597.

Romieu, I., J. A. Berlin, and G. Colditz. "Oral contraceptives and breast cancer. Review and meta-analysis." *Cancer 66* (1990): 2253–2263.

Rosenthal, M. Sara. *The Breast Sourcebook*, 2nd ed. New York City:McGraw-Hill, 1999.

Rundall, T., and W. Bruvold. "A meta-analysis of school-based smoking and alcohol use prevention programs." *Health Educational Quarterly* 15 (1988): 317–334.

Samet, J. M. "Indoor radon and lung cancer: risk or not? *Journal of the National Cancer Institute* 86 (1994): 1813–1814.

Saslow, D., et al. "American Cancer Society guideline for HPV Vaccine Use to Prevent Cervical Cancer and its Precursors." *CA: A Cancer Journal for Clinicians* 57 (2007): 7–28.

Schapiro, M. "Toxic inaction: why poisonous, unregulated chemicals end up in our blood." *Harper's Magazine* (2007): 78–83.

Schiffman, M. H., H. M. Bauer, R. N. Hoover, et al. "Epidemiologic evidence showing that human pappillomavirus infection causes most cervical intraepithelial neoplasia." *Journal of the National Cancer Institute* 85 (1993): 958–964.

Schiliro, T., C. Pignata, E. Fea, and G. Gilli. "Toxicity and estrogenic activity of a wastewater treatment plant in Northern Italy." *Archives of Environmental Contamination and Toxicology* 47 (2004): 456–462.

Scribner, J. D., and N. K. Mottett. "DDT acceleration of mammary gland tumors induced in the male Sprague-Dewey rate by 2-acetamio-phenanthrene." *Carcinogenesis* 2 (1981): 1236–1239.

Shames, L. S., M. T. Munekata, and M. C. Pike. "Re: Blood levels of organochlorine residues and risk of breast cancer." *Journal of the National Cancer Institute* 86 (1994): 1642–1643.

Shannon, H. S., et al. "Lung cancer and air pollution in an industrial city—a geographical analysis." *Canadian Journal of Public Health* 79 (1988): 255–259.

Shimikawa, T., P. Soblie, M. A. Carpenter, et al. "Dietary intake patterns and sociodemographic factors in the atherosclerosis risk in communities study." *Preventive Medicine* 12 (1994): 769–780.

Soto, Ana M., et al. "p-Nonyl-Phenol: An estrogenic xenobiotic released from 'modified' polystyrene." *Environmental Health Perspectives* 92 (1991): 167–173.

Steingraber, Sandra. *Living Downstream: An Ecologist Looks at Cancer and the Environment.* New York: Addison-Wesley, 1997.

Stern, R. S., et al. "Risk reduction for nonmelanoma skin cancer with childhood sunscreen use." *Arch Dermatol* 122 (1986): 537–545.

Subramanian, J., and R. Govindan. "Lung cancer in never smokers: a review." *Journal of Clinical Oncology* 25 (2007): 561–570.

Surgeon General. *The Health Consequences of Involuntary Smoking.* Washington, D.C.: U.S. Dept of Health and Human Services, 1986.

Swerdlow, A. J., J. English, and R. M. Mackie. "Benign nevi associated with high risk of cutaneous malignant melanoma." *Lancet* 11 (1984): 168–170.

Takkouche, B., et al. "Personal Use of Hair Dyes and Risk of Cancer: A Meta-analysis." *JAMA* (2005).

The Alpha-Tocopherol, Beta Caroten Cancer Prevention Study Group. "The effect of vitamin B and beta carotene on the incidence of lung cancer and other cancers in smokers." *New England Journal of Medicine* 330 (1994): 1029–1035.

The Pacific Northwest Pollution Prevention Resource Center. "Pollution Charges and Taxes." (2008) http://www.pprc.org.

The WHO Collaborative Study of Neoplasia and Steroid Contraceptives. "Depo-medroxyprogesterone acetate (DMPA) and risk of endometrial cancer." *International Journal of Cancer* 49 (1991): 186–190.

Theriault, G., M. Goldberg, A. B. Miller, et al. "Cancer risks associated with occupational exposure to magnetic fields among electric utility workers in Ontario and Quebec, Canada and France: 1970-1989." *American Journal of Epidemiology* 139 (1994): 550–572.

Thomas, D. B. "Oral contraceptives and breast cancer." *Journal of the National Cancer Institute* 85 (1993): 359–364.

Thompson, D., D. Kriebel, M. M. Quinn, et al. "Occupational exposure to metalworking fluids and risk of breast cancer among female autoworkers." *American Journal of Industrial Medicine* 47 (2005): 153–160.

Thompson, S. C., D. Jolley, and R. Marks. "Reduction of solar keratoses by regular sunscreen use." *New England Journal of Medicine* 329 (1993): 1147–1151.

Thornton, J. Chlorine, Human Health and the Environment: *The Breast Cancer Warning*. Washington, D.C.: Greenpeace, 1993.

Thune, Inger, et al. "Physical Activity and the Risk of Breast Cancer." *New England Journal of Medicine* 336 (1997): 1269–1275.

Ting, W., K. Schultz, N. N. Cac, et al. "Tanning bed exposure increases the risk of malignant melanoma." *International Journal of Dermatology* 46 (2007): 1253–1257.

Tomatis, L., A. Aitio, N. E. Day, E. Heseltine, et al. *Cancer: Causes, Occurrence and Control*. Lyon: IARC Scientific Publications No. 100, 1990.

U.S. Department of Health and Human Services. *Reducing the Health Consequences of Smoking: 25 Years of Progress*. A report of the Surgeon General. Rockville, MD: U.S. Department of Health and Human Services, Centre for Disease Control, Centre for Chronic Disease Prevention and Health Promotion, Office on Smoking and Health, 1989.

U.S. Department of Health and Human Services. *The Health Consequences of Smoking: Cancer*. A report of the Surgeon General. Rockville, MD: U.S. Department of Health and Human Services, Public Health Service, Office on Smoking and Health, 1982.

U.S. Department of Health and Human Services. *The Health Consequences of Smoking: Chronic Obstructive Lung Disease*. A report of the Surgeon General. Rockville, MD: U.S. Department of Health and Human Services, Public Health Service, Office on Smoking and Health, 1984.

U.S. Department of Health and Human Services. *The Health Consequences of Smoking: Cardiovascular Disease*. A report of the Surgeon General. Rockville, MD: U.S. Department of Health and Human Services, Public Health Service, Office on Smoking and Health, 1983.

U.S. Department of Health and Human Services and U.S. Environmental Protection Agency. *Respiratory Health Effects of Passive Smoking: Lung Cancer and Other Disorders.* The Report of the U.S. Environmental Protection Agency. Smoking and Control Monograph 4. NIH Publication No. 93-3605, 1993.

U.S. Public Health Service. "Even some exercise offers health benefits." *Prevention Report*, October/November 1994.

Upton, A. C., T. Kneip, and P. Toniolo. "Public health aspects of toxic chemical disposal sites." *Annual Review of Public Health* 10 (1989): 1–25.

Vineis, P., and L. Simonato. "Estimates of the proportion of bladder cancers attributable to occupation." *Scandinavian Journal of Work Environmental Health* 12 (1986): 55–60.

Vitasa, B. C., et al. "Association of non-melanoma skin cancer and actinic keratosis and cumulative solar ultraviolet exposure in Maryland waterman." *Cancer* 65 (1990): 2811–2817.

Von Grote, J., C. Hurlimann, M. Scheringer, K. Hungerbuhler. "Assessing occupational exposure to perchloroethylene in dry-cleaning." *Journal of Occupational Environmental Hygine* 3 (2006): 606–619.

Walker, A. I. T., et al. "The toxicology and pharmacodynamics of dieldrin: two year oral exposure of rats and dogs." *Toxicology and Applied Pharmacology* 15 (1969): 345–373.

Wasserman, M., et al. "Organochlorine compounds in neoplastic and adjacent apparently normal breast tissue." *Bulletin Environmental Contaminants and Toxicology* 15 (1976): 478–484.

Webster, T. "Dioxin and human health: a public health assessment of dioxin exposure in Canada." Unpublished manuscript. Boston: Boston University School of Public Health, 1994.

Westin, J. B., and E. Richter. "The Israeli breast cancer anomaly." *Ann New York Acad Sci* 609 (1990): 269–279.

Whitehead, M. *The Health Divide.* London: Health Education Council, 1987.

Wigle, D. T., R. M. Semenciw, K. Wilkins, et al. "Mortality study of Canadian male farm operators: non-Hodgkins lymphoma and agricultural practices in Saskatchewan." *Journal of the National Cancer Institute* 82 (1990): 575–582.

Wilson, P. D., K. H. Kaldby, and A. M. Kligman. "Ultraviolet light sensitivity and prolonged UVR-erythema." *J Invest Dermatol* 77 (1981): 434–436.

Windsor Air Quality Committee. "Windsor air quality study." Toronto; Science and Technology Branch, Ministry of Environment and Energy, 1994.

Wolff, M. S., P. G. Toniolo, E. W. Lee, et al. "Blood levels of organochlorine residues and risk of breast cancer." *Journal of the National Cancer Institute* 85 (1993): 648–652.

World Health Organization. Ionizing Rafiation in Our Environment. (2008) www.who.int/ionizing_radiation/env/en.

World Health Organization/International Agency for Research on Cancer. *World Cancer Report*. Bernard W. Stewart and Paul Kleihues, eds. (2003).

Zeka, A., E. A. Eisen, D. Kriebel, et al. "Risk of upper aerodigestive tract cancers in a case-cohort study of autoworkers exposed to metalworking fluids." *Occupational and Environmental Medicine* 61 (2004): 426–431.

INDEX

dietary fat, 21, 40, 43, 45
differentiated, 17–18
dioxin, 121
dry-cleaning, 123, 174, 178
dysplasia, 94

E

education, income, and cancer risk, 23
electromagnetic fields (EMF), 118, 126,
   137–138, 144
environmental carcinogens, 141
environmental estrogens, 151
estrogen, 23, 39, 44, 57, 87, 97–104,
   121, 142, 144, 148, 163, 168

F

familial adenomatous polyposis, 85
fat, 39–41, 46
fiber, 12, 25, 41–43, 46–48, 86, 137
fruits and vegetables, 41
food labels, 48
food made in China, 160
food packaging and storage, 106–108

G

genes, 12, 81–87, 132, 159
genes and infectious diseases, 81
genes, common cancer
   BRCA1, 83, 87, 89
   BRCA2, 83, 87, 89
   p16, 83
   MLH1, 83
   MSH2, 83
   MSH6, 83
   PMS2, 83
genetic counseling, 85, 86–89
genetic discrimination, 90
genetic testing, 82–91
grading, cell, 18, 52
Great Lakes, 139, 141, 163–182
Great Lakes Basin ecosystem, 162–164
Great Lakes Water Quality Agreement,
   165–166, 180–182

H

hair dyes, 101–102
hereditary breast-ovarian cancer
   syndrome, 87
hereditary nonpolyposis colon cancer
   syndrome, 85
high risk jobs, possible, 137–138
HIV, 91–93, 104
HIV/AIDS, 91–93
HIV-related cancers, 92
   Kaposi's sarcoma, 92
   non-Hodgkin's lymphoma, 92–93, 120
   cervical cancer, 28, 43, 92–94
home-cleaning products, 104
Home Safe Home, (Dadd), 104
hormone-containing medications, 102
human papillomavirus (HPV), 30, 91–94
hybrid cars, 155

I J

infectious diseases, 91, 94
Insider, The, 34
in situ, 17
invasive, 17, 91, 169, 177, 179
iodine, 44, 114, 142–143
ionizing radiation, 109
iron, 43

K

Kaposi's sarcoma, 92
known cancer agents, 135–137

L

legumes, 41, 47
*Living Downstream: An Ecologist Looks at
   Cancer and the Environment,*
   (Steingraber), 44, 139, 147, 150

M

man-made sources of radiation, 115
meat, 23, 42–54, 86, 157, 159
melanoma, 69–72, 75–78
metalworking fluids, 122, 127, 135
methylene chloride, 104, 122–123